Understanding Stammering or Stuttering

Understanding Stammering or Stuttering

A Guide for Parents, Teachers and Other Professionals

Elaine Kelman and Alison Whyte

Foreword by Michael Palin

Jessica Kingsley *Publishers*
London and Philadelphia

Children's artwork has been reproduced with kind permission from the children and their families.

First published in 2012
by Jessica Kingsley Publishers
116 Pentonville Road
London N1 9JB, UK
and
400 Market Street, Suite 400
Philadelphia, PA 19106, USA

www.jkp.com

Library of Congress Cataloging in Publication Data
Kelman, Elaine.
 Understanding stammering or stuttering : guide for parents, teachers and other professionals / Elaine
Kelman and Alison Whyte ; foreword by Michael Palin.
   p. cm.
 Includes bibliographical references and index.
 ISBN 978-1-84905-268-9 (alk. paper)
 1. Stuttering. 2. Speech disorders. I. Whyte, Alison. II. Title.
 RC424.K427 2012
 616.85'54--dc23
                              2012013481

British Library Cataloguing in Publication Data
A CIP catalogue record for this book is available from the British Library

ISBN 978 1 84905 268 9
eISBN 978 0 85700 543 4

Printed and bound in Great Britain

To all the children, young people and families
who have taught us so much

CONTENTS

FOREWORD

As long as I knew my father, and probably for many years before that, he suffered from a stammer. It was at times so severe that he would just give up trying to say what he wanted to say. And there was a lot he wanted to say. Like many people who stammer he was bright and intelligent. He had a good sense of humour, but telling jokes was a no-go area for him, requiring a precision and fluency that continually let him down. Looking back now, I can see that the flashes of temper that were also characteristic of him must have come from living in a constant state of frustration, let down by something we all take for granted, the gift of fluent speech.

In 1985 John Cleese, with whom I'd worked on the Monty Python films and television shows, asked if I could draw on my father's experience to help him create a character with a stammer for a film that eventually became *A Fish Called Wanda*. The resulting film was a great success and I received all sorts of feedback from people concerned with the rights and wrongs of portraying a character who stammers in a comedy.

One approach was from a man called Travers Reid who was a friend and supporter of the work of a formidable speech therapist called Lena Rustin. Lena's particular area of interest was stammering in children. We met together and for the first time I heard some sensible talk about stammering. How it might begin, how it could be detected and how it could be managed to reduce its crippling effect on the confidence of the youngster. This was fascinating and inspiring, not just knowing that children could be helped but that lives, like that of my father, need not have been consumed with frustration and tension. I knew that I had to do whatever I could to make sure that Lena Rustin's therapy was made available to as many children as possible.

So, in 1993, with help from many people, not least Travers Reid and the family of Gerald Ronson, the Michael Palin Centre for Stammering Children opened, and from an initial staff of one and a half a week, it has grown to 11 speech and language therapists in a comfortable, spacious, well-equipped home in Finsbury in London. It is seen as a centre of excellence and has been the model for a similar centre in the north of England. Sadly, Lena Rustin didn't live long enough to see the Centre flourishing as it is now. Elaine Kelman, the co-author of this book, is one of the longest serving of the dedicated and enormously talented team recruited by Lena, and I can think of no one better qualified to write on the subject of stammering.

'Understanding' is one of the most important words in the treatment of stammering. At a literal level it means understanding what someone is trying to say, but at a much deeper level it is about understanding why and how they are unable to say it. There are many other questions too. Why does it affect some children and not others, why is it proportionally more common in boys than girls, why can it disappear only to recur years later?

The other important word, which to my mind typifies Lena Rustin's approach and characterises the treatment at the Michael Palin Centre is 'listening'. There is no 'one size fits all' therapy for stammering. There is no magic wand, or pill or potion which can make dysfluency vanish. Each child must be listened to individually. The family must be listened to as well. Parents and siblings can provide valuable clues as to the origins of the stammer. Listening requires patience, a quality that Elaine and her colleagues have in abundance. It can be a long-term process, but it must never be rushed. Treating a stammer is about the relief of pressure, not its application. But it does work. I have been greatly moved by meeting parents who come to the Centre and who see an improvement, sometimes a dramatic improvement, in the fluency of their children. Their relief and joy is palpable. Very often the key to unlock the problem has been the shared experience of meeting other parents whose children have similar problems.

Part of my own helplessness about my father's stammer is that we never talked about it. It was seen as an affliction that had no cure. Drawing attention to it would only make the pain worse. In our household there was no listening and therefore no understanding. Mercifully, things are different now. Thanks in part to the success of the film, The King's Speech, and television documentaries showing the work of the Centre, the subject of stammering is no longer taboo.

Elaine Kelman and Alison Whyte's book is written in the spirit of openness and participation. It covers most of the things you ever wanted to know about stammering but never dared ask. Above all, it puts the voice of the young person at the heart of the book. As the authors say in their introduction, 'the child who stammers is the only expert.'

Of course I wish a book like this had been available in the dark years of the past when stammering was seen as a guilty secret, an expression of limited ability, something which you had to suffer in silence. But I'm very proud to have been associated, through the Centre, with such a complete change in attitude. To all those who stammer, who are parents or teachers, or sons and daughters of people who stammer, this book will bring hope and comfort. And yes, help to transform lives too.

Michael Palin
London, March 2012

ACKNOWLEDGEMENTS

We would like to thank the trustees of Action for Stammering Children for all they have done to help children who stammer and their families, and in particular for supporting the writing of this book.

Also Frances Cook and Diana de Grunwald for their wisdom, advice, support and unerring 'red pen' in the preparation of the manuscript.

The professional advice includion here is the culmination of over two decades of team work at the Michael Palin Centre and we want to thank the therapists there, acknowledging the pioneering work of the late Lena Rustin, perpetuated and developed by Willie Botterill and the rest of the team. Their creativity, hard work and openness to new ideas has helped the Centre's work to maintain consistently high standards of care for all those they seek to help.

Finally, we would like to thank the children, young people and their families from whom we have learned so much over the years and especially those whose words are included in the pages that follow.

Elaine Kelman and Alison Whyte

INTRODUCTION

Why did you pick up this book? Would you like to find out how to help someone you know who has a stammer? Perhaps you have a child who stammers. The stammer may have begun quite suddenly – even overnight – for no apparent reason. Or it may have appeared gradually, and at first you weren't worried. Perhaps your child's stammer seems to be entrenched and you are beginning to feel anxious about what the future may bring. Or perhaps your child has been stammering for years. He may have had speech and language therapy, and nothing seems to help.

Parents have been contacting the Michael Palin Centre for many years. Some are seeking information, reassurance, or practical help and advice. Some feel powerless; they don't know where to turn. Some are wracked with guilt because they believe they have done something to cause their child to stammer. Some have been given misleading information by professionals or well-meaning friends and relatives.

The questions parents ask are endless:

- Why is this happening?

- Did I cause it to happen?

- Will it just stop if I do nothing?

- Is it a stammer or a stutter?

- Should I mention it to him?

- Should I try to help him when he's stuck?

- What have I done wrong?

- Why does it come and go?

- Is it because we're so busy?

- Why does he not stammer when he sings?

- Is he copying someone else who stammers?

- How will he cope at school?

- Will he be bullied?

- What about oral exams?

- Will he ever get a job?

- What can I do?

- Where can I get some help?

Whoever you are, whatever the reason for your interest in stammering, we hope this book will help. As a parent you may feel lost, worried about your child's future, unable to chart the way ahead. We hope that this book will help you to understand what stammering is, and how it affects children, their parents and the rest of the family. We hope you will find in it useful advice about how to support your child as he navigates his way through school, within friendships and through social situations, and where you can find help.

Stammering is a very complicated problem because it appears in many different forms. It can change from one moment to the next, or one day to another for no apparent reason. It can vanish for weeks or months only to reappear. It can wreak havoc on the lives of some children or it can be a quirky feature that never really gets in the way.

Each child is differently affected so we need to treat him as an individual, taking care to work out the best way to help him and his family. There is no 'one size fits all' therapy for children who stammer and neither can this book be 'one size fits all'. We are trying to cover the whole range of possible scenarios that children and their families may face.

In so doing, there is a risk. Have you ever visited the doctor and been told that you might have a certain medical condition, then gone away to look it up in a medical encyclopaedia or on the web? This can be a mistake because you will read about all the worst-case scenarios and the worst possible outcomes, and thoroughly frighten yourself.

This book is for the parent who is curious about their child's stammering, but not overly concerned, as well as parents who are beside themselves with worry. And we don't want you to think that every child who stammers will face all the issues described here. We have tried to talk about them all in case they are a problem; they are not a foregone conclusion.

This book is called *Understanding Stammering and Stuttering*. These are simply two words that describe the same thing. The word stammering is more widely used in the UK, while the term stuttering is more common in America.

In the book we use the word stammer to describe what happens when someone is trying to speak but no words come out. He may get stuck, he may repeat a word or sound, or stretch the word out. He may stop talking or change the word he was about to say, he may contort his face or body in an effort to speak. All of this is part of the stammer or stutter.

One of the interesting facts about stammering is that it affects more boys than girls. You are probably five times more likely to be reading this book because you know a boy who stammers. For this reason, we mainly refer to 'he' in this book.

You may have picked up this book because you are looking for some expert information and advice. But who is the expert on stammering? The speech and language therapist who has worked with children who stammer for many years? The parent who has cared for the child all his life? Or the child himself?

The child who stammers is the only expert. Only he can tell you what it feels like to know what he wants to say, but because of a blockage in his mouth he is unable to get it out. Only he can describe the pressure he feels when he has been asked a question and all eyes are on him, but when he opens his mouth to respond there is only silence. Only he can tell you how frustrating it is to have a great story to tell, but not to be able to tell it. While we are able to concentrate solely on what we want to say, he can feel exhausted by having to think about the very act of speaking all day and every day.

In the following pages, the real experts – children and young people who stammer – will answer some of the questions. You will hear their voices loud and clear. Their names have been changed to respect their right to anonymity. You will also hear the voices of parents of children who stammer, who will share their worries and their joy when their children overcome some of the difficulties that stammering presents. You will also hear from speech and language therapists at the Michael Palin Centre, who have worked for many years at the largest centre specialising in supporting children who stammer in the UK.

The authors of this book are a speech and language therapist and a journalist who is a parent of a young man who stammers. We write as one voice but the knowledge and experience of both influences what we say.

We have learned what we know from our experience here in the UK. And we have also learned from our international professional colleagues. So most of the information here will apply to children who stammer and their families, wherever they may be in the world. The chapter on information and resources focuses on therapy that is available and we have tried to make this international, but there will be differences according to where you are. So we have signposted where you can get more information, typically online, that is relevant to your location.

We want the voices of children and young people to be clearly heard in this book so we have begun each section with their quotes. We also place great importance on listening to parents. Parents know their own child. They know what helps and what doesn't. Speech and language therapists tailor the knowledge parents already have to help them support their child. Our mantra is 'Parents know, they just don't know that they know.' We have found that once parents learn to trust their own instincts and knowledge their confidence will grow.

We ask you to listen to the voices of children and their parents, the true experts, who have taught us so much.

WHAT YOUNG PEOPLE SAY
ABOUT STAMMERING

'Having a stammer makes talking really hard work.'

Hanna, 12

'It makes me feel frustrated, angry, upset – why should I be treated differently just because I've got a stammer?'

Amir, 14

'Sometimes I feel lonely coz I think I'm the only one in the world who has this problem.'

Josh, 8

'When people finish my sentences for me, I get really annoyed coz they think they know what I want to say – but when they get it wrong I have to start all over again.'

Moishe, 14

'People who stammer aren't stupid – we just need a bit more time to get our words out.'

Rachel, 9

'Sometimes I want to say something and I can't say a single word. The people around me don't even know that I'm trying to talk, that I'm trying to force out what I want to say and by the time I get it out they'll have already have moved on. It's so frustrating.'

Joe, 15

'Having a stammer is not a very good thing to have coz you don't join in on any activities that require speaking and you feel left out.'

Wayne, 9

'I can't do presentations; I can't do things like talking in front of people. I can't even talk to a whole group of people and it also makes me not answer questions at school when I know lots of them.'

Ahmed, 10

'I like to think I'm a normal person, but people don't see it that way when I open my mouth to speak and the words just won't come out.'

Ryan, 16

'People do tend to think of me as different to everyone else coz I have a stammer but then everybody is different in their own way. People can make a big deal out of it but personally I just roll with it.'

Zac, 15

Chapter 1

STAMMERING

THE FACTS

'I imagine my stammer like a brick wall because it's hard to get things out.'

Charlotte, 14

'I've always imagined it as bars across my mouth stopping me from speaking.'

Max, 20

Stammering is a very complicated and confusing problem. No two stammers are the same, and a stammer can change over time. So what exactly is a stammer?

WHAT YOU SEE

'I sometimes get completely blocked around my throat and the words get stuck, and a sound like 'w' gets blocked around my lips, my shoulders get tense and my eyes shut.'

Yousef, 15

Although stammering varies from child to child, it has some common features. A child may:

- repeat whole words (e.g. 'and…and, and then I left')

- repeat parts of words (e.g. 'b-be-because I c-c-c-c-can')

- prolong or stretch out certain sounds (e.g. 'sssssssometimes I g…ooooooo…out')

- 'block', where the mouth is in position but no sound comes out

- tense up his face, especially the muscles around the eyes, nose, lips or neck (some children appear to have facial contortions – they may blink or twitch or use their tongue or lips to try to force the words out)

- stiffen up his whole body or part of his body just before he speaks

- adopt extra body movements as he tries to 'push' the word out (he may stamp his feet, thump his chest, tap his thigh or slap a desk or table)

- display a disrupted breathing pattern (e.g. he may hold his breath while speaking or take a very deep intake of breath before speaking).

Fluency seems to break down more frequently when children try to use longer words and to form more complicated sentences. Stammering is more likely to happen at the beginning of a sentence or phrase and with less familiar words.

Children often have several of the features listed above, and they may stammer in different ways in different settings and at different times. The flow of speech is generally bumpy and interrupted, which may upset the child and his parents or friends.

The visual signs that often accompany stammering can be very distressing to parents – especially if the child appears to be really struggling to get his words out, and when people are waiting to hear what he has to say. The temptation to help the child to finish his sentence can be almost overwhelming.

Despite the fact that children can appear to be in some distress while they are trying to speak – opening and closing their mouths, twitching or contorting their faces or bodies – it can sometimes feel even worse for the parents who are watching. Some children say they are concentrating on getting their words out, that they are not always feeling as anxious inside as they appear on the outside.

Some children say that the body movements and other physical traits they have are part of the stammer itself. Sometimes they may not even be very aware that their bodies are moving, and consequently may not realise how they appear to others while they are stammering.

Stammering often changes over time, with various features appearing or disappearing. A child who used to stammer at the beginning of words may suddenly start to block. A child who used to slap his thigh while trying to speak may suddenly stop doing it – or else switch to something different, such as closing his eyes while speaking.

WHAT YOU DON'T SEE

> 'It's quite hard a lot of the time coz you don't say what you want to say and you have to, like, always keep on changing what you're about to say to avoid stammering.'
>
> Steven, 9

Sometimes a child will try to hide or reduce his stammer. He may:

- pretend that he has forgotten what he was going to say

- switch to another word when he begins to stammer (e.g. 'Please can I have a ch- ch- ch-…a vanilla ice cream')

- avoid speaking in front of other people

- not put up his hand or ask any questions in class

- opt out of activities that involve speaking

- display behaviour to draw attention away from the stammer – such as clowning around in class.

Some children say that they speak much less than they would like to, for instance they may hold back in a group, or not tell a joke or a story because it would take too long or it wouldn't come out right. This can be very damaging to their confidence.

As they get older, children can become very skilled at changing what they were planning to say in order to avoid an approaching stammer – so skilful that people don't realise they are doing it. Sometimes their speech becomes convoluted and difficult to follow as a result.

Some older children and teenagers are so adept at managing their stammer that they appear to 'surf' their sentences – pausing to take breath at certain points, letting several words rush out at once.

Some children manage to hide the stammer so successfully that people don't even know that they stammer. They may just be seen as 'the shy girl' or 'the quiet boy' at the back of the class. In fact, they may be anything but shy or quiet. This is why children who stammer sometimes say they are not seen as they really are.

The iceberg

The late American therapist Joseph Sheehan described a stammer as being like an iceberg. This is an analogy that we still use in therapy to illustrate how much of the stammer is unseen by the onlooker. We know that there are two parts to an iceberg – the part you see above the waterline and the part under the water that you don't see – by far the larger of the two.

The same applies to stammering. Some of it you see – the blocking, the expression on the face, the body movements. But there can be very much more that is hidden – emotions, physical sensations and the things the child is doing to manage the stammer or hide it. There are two examples of icebergs drawn and illustrated by children on the next page.

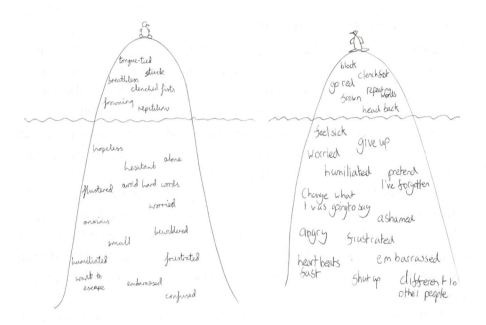

Drawings of an iceberg by Jon aged 17 and Chris aged 11

QUESTIONS AND ANSWERS ABOUT STAMMERING

Stammer or stutter?

The two words mean exactly the same thing but 'stammer' is the term normally used in Britain while the word 'stutter' is more common in the United States.

Do children stammer throughout the world?

Yes. Stammering can be found all over the world – in all countries, and among all races, religions and languages. It affects people from all kinds of backgrounds.

How many children stammer?

About 5 per cent of children experience some difficulty with their fluency at some point in their lives. Most children will achieve normal fluency with or without help, but about one in every 100 children will continue to stammer into adulthood.

Have children always stammered?

In his fascinating book about the history of stammering, David Compton says the first documented reference to stammering was 2500 years ago, by the Chinese poet Laotze (Compton 1993). Stammering was also known to the ancient Greeks – Heroditus wrote about it around 400 BCE.

Over the ages, stammering has been variously described as an anatomical disorder, a disease, a psychiatric illness, an anomaly of brain functioning and an emotional disturbance.

In the middle ages, stammering was seen as a personality disorder and people who stammered were thought to be possessed by the devil. The possessed person was made to drink garlic and vinegar in order to vomit out the stammer. In the 1700s people who stammered had their tongues severed, pierced with hot needles or had pieces of their tongue removed.

Different 'cures' were applied throughout Europe during the 1800s and people who stammered were flogged, had leeches applied to their lips, were forced to eat laxatives or were given electric shocks to the spine.

In the early 1800s, a 'stuttering clinic' was founded in New York by a Dr Yates. He instructed the person with a stammer to keep the tip of his tongue on the palate while speaking – almost an impossible task. This 'cure' was later exposed as utterly useless.

Probably the most famous person to stammer in England was King George VI, father of Elizabeth II, and the subject of the award-winning film *The King's Speech* in 2011. His courageous and public struggle to speak in radio broadcasts and in front of thousands of spectators inspired many people who stammer.

So stammering has been documented throughout history – it is by no means a new phenomenon.

Do both girls and boys stammer?

In early childhood, there are almost as many girls as boys who stammer, but this changes over time. It seems that girls are more likely to overcome a stammer than boys. By the age of 10, about five times as many boys have a stammer.

When does stammering begin?

> We first noticed it at the age of 3, at preschool. When he did try and speak there was first sound repetition, m-m-m-m-mummy. His pronunciation wasn't always spot on and he was always quite rushed to get it out. He'd ask, 'Can I do that, can I do that?' At that stage we didn't even know it was stammering, we just thought it was part of his speech development.
>
> *Mother of 12-year-old boy*

> She used very flowery sentences very early on and her speech was very fluent when she was very young. We used to say, 'Tell us *The Owl and the Pussycat*' and she could recite the whole thing. We first noticed the stammer when she was about 5. She started to stumble with words a little bit. It has deteriorated since…it's the b, the g, the m… Now there are lots of head movements and lots of blinking, too much pressure, lots of tension in her neck as though she's blowing up a balloon, really holding on to things quite hard.
>
> *Mother of 14-year-old girl*

Many children go through a stage when they stumble over words. This stumbling phase usually happens when they are learning to speak, and can last for a few weeks or months before the child becomes fluent again.

Stammering generally starts when a child's language is developing rapidly between the ages of 2 and 5. It has been suggested that the dramatic increase in language skills that children develop at this age may 'overload' the system. Some parents describe this by saying, 'His brain is going faster than his mouth.'

Parents often tell us that when children try to use complicated language they stammer more. Their fluency may also break down when they are being asked to explain things, or if they are excited about retelling a story, or trying to speak very quickly.

Parents sometimes link the onset of stammering to a time when the child's language development speeded up, or believe his fluency began to falter just when his reading was taking off.

For some children, the stammer starts gradually: it comes and goes, and seems to be a part of a child's effort to use more and more words. For other children, stammering can begin quite suddenly, almost overnight. This can be very worrying, for both the child and for his family. Sometimes the stammer can disappear just as quickly as it came.

Does stammering affect intelligence?

'If someone said that I'm inferior to them because of my talking, then well obviously I disagree because at school I'd like to think I'm one of the bright ones.'

Dan, 16

There is no truth in the idea that people who stammer are not as intelligent as people who don't. Stammering is a speech disorder that has no connection with a person's intellect. People who stammer show the same range of intelligence as the rest of the population.

Why does the stammer come and go?

'I don't think I'm any different to anyone else, I just go through bad patches and good patches and when I go through the bad patches I'm a bit quiet and when I go through the good patches I'm pretty good, pretty loud.'

Abassi, 9

Stammering can be unpredictable. A child can stammer severely at certain times, and at other times hardly at all. The stammer can vary in severity from day to day, week to week, month to month. Some researchers think the variability in stammering may be related to spurts in development.

The fact that children with stammers are sometimes fluent can deter parents from seeking help. Some children can go for weeks or months without stammering, and their parents think the stammer has gone – only for it to start again for no apparent reason.

Children can stammer more at certain times of the day (especially when they are tired), in certain situations (when they are competing with others to speak), when they are at a significant stage of their lives (when they start at a new school) or when they are unwell.

Parents can find the fluctuations in fluency bewildering.

> Some members of the family are very sceptical about his stammer. They seem to think it doesn't really exist. They say things like 'Well I've never really noticed it' or 'He seems to me to speak normally'. This is upsetting because it suggests that they think we are suffering from some kind of neurosis, projecting a problem onto our child that isn't really there.

Mother of teenage boy

The fact that stammering can fluctuate so much can make it incredibly frustrating for the person who stammers. One student who thought he had learned to live with his stammer told us that he was so overwhelmed when he had to do a presentation while at university that he simply ran out of the room.

Why does he not stammer when he sings?

It is curious that a child who struggles to speak is able to sing fluently. A number of people who stammer have become famous singers – most recently, Gareth Gates of the UK version of *Pop Idol* fame.

We think that this is because singing involves a different part of the brain to speaking. The combination of the melody (which comes from the right side of the brain) and the speech (which comes from the left side of the brain) results in fluency.

Many years ago, people tried to use a singing therapy to treat stammering, but nobody wants to have to sing everything; in any case, whenever someone stops singing and starts speaking, the stammer usually returns.

Does stammering affect a child's ability to read and write?

We have often been asked whether there is a connection between a stammer and a child's ability to read and write. Children who stammer are no more likely to have reading and writing difficulties than children who are fluent speakers.

Some children who stammer may also have dyslexia, but there is no evidence that the two difficulties are linked. Stammering may deter a child from reading aloud, but this does not mean there's an underlying problem with his literacy skills.

Will he grow out of his stammer?

Research and our experience help us to understand that children who are most likely to grow out of stammering are children who:

- do not have any relatives who stammer

- are girls

- have relatives who stammered when they were children but grew out of it

- seem to be improving

- have been stammering for less than a year

- are not aware of the stammer or who are not anxious about it

- have parents who are not worried about the stammer

- had clear pronunciation around the time when the stammering started.

There doesn't seem to be a link between the way a child stammers, how severely he stammers and whether the child is likely to stammer into adulthood. Many of the children who stammer severely when they are young will grow out of it.

So if you have a son, if other members of your family stammer, if your child has been stammering for over a year, if his speech was unclear when he started to stammer, if he is aware of his stammer and is anxious about it and you also are worried…get some help. Ask to have him assessed by a speech and language therapist.

The longer a child has been stammering, the less likely he is to grow out it. He can still benefit hugely from treatment, but the difficulty is unlikely to resolve without help.

Do parents cause stammering?

> Of course you worry that it's your fault…maybe if we'd nipped it in the bud, if we'd gone to therapy earlier, if we hadn't been out at work so much, if he'd eaten a different diet. And why didn't we notice it before and do something about it?
>
> *Mother of 12-year-old boy*

Nan Bernstein Ratner (2010, p.237), an eminent authority in the field of stammering, wrote: 'It is sometimes both amazing and saddening for me to talk to families who describe a fairly clear pattern of stuttering inheritance, with grandparents, uncles, cousins and so on, but still ask "What did we do to cause this problem?"'

Parents do not cause their children to stammer, but many parents think they are to blame. The fact that we don't fully understand why people stammer means that there is lots of scope for speculation. Parents say they are often asked what they think has caused their child to stammer. The very question can induce feelings of guilt.

Recent research shows that the brains of children who stammer may differ slightly from the brains of other children (see the next section on 'Causes of stammering').

Could a stammer be caused by a traumatic event?

At the Michael Palin Centre we are often asked whether a child's stammer could have been caused by a trauma or an upset in the family. There is no research to back this up, but there are many anecdotes linking stammering to events – the arrival of a new baby, starting school or nursery, being severely told off, getting ill or having an accident.

However, few children grow up without experiencing an upset of some kind. Most children have siblings, go to nurseries, get shouted at and fall off their bikes – and they don't stammer. Rather than being the cause of the stammer, a significant event in the life of a child whose speech was already vulnerable may have acted as a trigger. Or it may have been a coincidence that the stammer began at around the time the event took place.

Can a stammer be 'cured'?

The word 'cure' makes stammering sound like an illness, which it is not. And no, there is no quick fix or cure. But a stammer can improve and many children stammer less as they get older.

However, our experience at the Michael Palin Centre tells us that the longer a child has been stammering, the less likely it is that the stammer will disappear entirely. Children who stammer can greatly improve their fluency using many different techniques, and a child's ability to manage the stammer can increase over time. A stammer need not limit a child's potential.

CAUSES OF STAMMERING

Speaking fluently is actually very complicated. Those of us who don't stammer take our ability to speak for granted. Fluent speech involves thinking of the right words, forming grammatical sentences, and getting them to come out of your mouth in the right order and with the right pronunciation in a fraction of a second.

Research shows that stammering may be caused by 'mismatches' in a child's speech and language skills (Beal 2011). He may be able to understand very complicated language but he may have difficulty putting his own thoughts into words. Or he may have a wide vocabulary but his ability to construct sentences may still be developing. He may find it hard to pronounce certain sounds or he may not be able to find the words to express just what he wants to say.

If one aspect of a child's speech and language ability is out of line with the rest, this may cause his fluency to break down. These problems can be quite slight and may only show up clearly when assessed in a speech and language therapy clinic.

It's a boy thing

We already know that stammering affects boys more than girls. Although the number of boys and girls who show signs of stammering under the age of 5 is roughly similar, by the age of 10, around five times as many boys as girls still stammer.

It's genetic

We also know that stammering tends to run in families. Ask someone who stammers if another person in the family has a stammer; they will almost always say 'yes'. We also know that if a child's relatives stammered into adulthood, he is more likely to do the same. Equally, if other family members grew out of the stammer, the child is likely to do so too.

In 1983, research in the US established that the incidence of stammering among the parents, children or siblings of people who stammer was three times higher than in the general population (Andrews *et al.* 1983). Studies have also shown that there are few sets of identical twins where only one stammers (Compton 1993). Either both do, or neither does.

Research indicates that up to 70 per cent of people who stammer may have an inherited predisposition towards stammering (Yairi and Ambrose 2005). And in 2010 a study was published indicating which genes might be involved in stammering (Kang, Riazuddin and Mundorff 2010).

Researchers are trying to establish which genes are involved because gene therapy can sometimes be used to 'block' gene activity in order to prevent transmission through families. But the gene activity that seems to be involved in stammering is also connected to a number of other essential functions, so blocking it is not an option.

The brain

'People don't realise it's just a mind trick, something that happens, we aren't actually retarded or stupid or can't think straight.'

Hassan, 12

'They do need to be aware that I can't help it. It's just my, it's just like how I was born, with a stammer.'

Sean, 10

The latest research shows that stammering may be related to the structure of the brain or the way it is working (Beal 2011). For some time it has been known that the brain activity of adults who stammer differs from that of fluent speakers. Brain scans show that in a fluent speaker, activity is predominantly in only one hemisphere of the brain, (typically on the left side). In people who stammer there is simultaneous activity on both sides of the brain. However, these findings are not conclusive; it is possible that the extra brain activity may have been caused by the stammer itself.

In young children, the wiring of the brain is still 'plastic' and can 'rewire' itself, either naturally or through therapy, so that the stammer resolves in time. This may explain why most children who start to stammer become fluent as they grow older. Our brains become more 'hard-wired' over time, which is why it's good to seek help as soon as possible.

If researchers could look at the brain function of young children they may be able to find out if their brains differ, either in their structure or in the way they function, before the stammer emerges. It would then be possible to deduce exactly what is causing the stammer. However, brain function can only be examined by using functional magnetic resonance imaging or fMRI – an expensive and potentially distressing procedure. It would be neither practical nor ethical to scan the brains of very young children.

'Glitches' in a child's developing system

Learning to talk involves coordinating signals in the brain to select and form words, shape them into sentences, then to articulate the sounds using the speech organs and muscles in the mouth, face and throat.

This complex system is constantly developing and, at times, various aspects of this system may not work in synchrony with other aspects. 'Glitches' can occur in this complicated process. Researchers think that these glitches are very typical in any child's developing system, but they normally resolve themselves spontaneously (Coutler, Anderson and Conture 2009).

Children who stammer have glitches that may need some help to be sorted out. The good news is that as the developing brain is 'plastic' or soft-wired, these glitches may be temporary and can be resolved in many cases. But this underlines the importance of getting help early whenever possible.

It is interesting to think about whether we can change the way the brain functions once we are older and 'hard-wired'. Researchers have found that if a person practises a particular skill for many hours, a scan will show actual changes in the brain function (Bernstein Ratner 2010). So a footballer practising penalty kicks over and over again changes what is happening in his brain. It is like he is pre-programming his brain to kick the ball in exactly the right way. This leads us to believe that any practising a child does with his speech can help to manage the 'glitches' in the brain.

Our therapy with older children therefore usually involves, amongst other things, some kind of speech technique that children practise very regularly until they can do it fairly naturally. That makes it sound easy. It isn't. It's very hard work and like any practice – be it piano scales or back exercises – it becomes boring and irritating. So this is not a magic solution, but one component of helping the child to feel a bit more in control some of the time.

WHAT AFFECTS A STAMMER?
The child's environment

> In the summer holidays it continued to get worse, and I thought 'It's all the excitement, late nights and going on holiday.' Then Christmas came, and I thought 'It's because of Christmas,' but in fact her stammer has deteriorated and now I know it's because she's having to work so hard to communicate.
>
> *Mother of 14-year-old girl*

'Having a stammer makes me feel nervous in some situations, for example if I'm on the bus and I'm being put on the spot, like having to buy a ticket. If I'm being hurried along in some situations I will find it much harder to answer the question because all that extra pressure has just been put on to you – it isn't very helpful to me at all.'

John, 13

Some children are more affected by their environment than others. Some children who stammer tell us that their fluency is affected by who they are with and how confident they feel in a particular place, setting or environment. It may be better or worse at home or at school, with family, friends or strangers, in familiar or unfamiliar surroundings. The social environment doesn't cause stammering, but it can have a big impact on the person who stammers.

The child who stammers may find it harder to be fluent when trying to speak at the same speed as other people, to join in rapid conversations or to form long or complicated sentences. It can be worse when children feel under pressure or they are put on the spot. They may find the busy pace of life that is normal in many families more difficult to cope with. Always having to hurry up can have a negative impact on the stammer.

The child's personality

> 'I don't think stammering makes anybody different to anybody else, it's just part of their personality and they should be treated the same as people who can speak fluently.'
>
> Philip, 10

People who stammer have many different types of personality. However, children who are very sensitive, who worry about making mistakes, who are perfectionists, who lack confidence, or who are impatient may find having a stammer especially hard to cope with.

Children who are naturally confident or who care less about how others see them may struggle less. But it's important to remember that children can grow in confidence: a shy child can blossom as an adolescent, and a nervous teenager can become a successful and self-assured adult.

The key thing to remember is that with love, support and encouragement even the most anxious child who stammers can gain confidence and reach his full potential.

How we respond

'My family try to teach me to just calm down and just take things extremely slowly because the slower I speak the less I seem to stammer.'

John, 13

'Sometimes someone might have said something to me that they thought was fine but I didn't really like it, like if they asked me what my name was and I took a long time to say it and they said, "Have you forgotten it?" as a joke, I might get a bit upset.'

Sean, 10

The way we respond to a child who is stammering has a major impact on the child, on his confidence and on his ability to speak.

We know that the way we feel can affect our speech – if we are nervous or excited we may speed up and stumble more, if we are really angry our minds can go blank. We can become 'speechless' with rage.

Parents usually tell us that their children stammer more when they are excited, anxious or self-conscious. Interestingly, while some children stammer more when they are angry or upset, others are more fluent. Some children don't stammer when they shout.

Children and young people who stammer have told us that the way people respond to their stammering can induce feelings of anxiety or anger. That's why it's very important to talk to your child about how he wants you to react while he is stammering. Later in this book we will explain a bit more about how best to approach this.

While it's good to praise a child when his speech is fluent, there is a fine line to walk. Too much praise for fluency can result in the child thinking that his stammer is a very bad thing and it is not acceptable to his parents. While praising a child when he is fluent will help to build his confidence, he also needs to know that he is loved and accepted, stammer and all.

SUCCESS STORIES

A quick look through the roll call of famous people who have stammered is a powerful reminder that stammering need not be an obstacle to a successful and fulfilling life.

Isacc Newton, who discovered the law of gravity, had a stammer, as did Charles Darwin, who formulated the theory of evolution. The politician Ed Balls stammers as did Aneurin Bevin and Winston Churchill.

The list of famous writers who stammered or still do includes Erasmus, Charles Lamb, Lewis Carroll, Somerset Maugham, Aldous Huxley, Kenneth Tynan, Margaret Drabble, Philip Larkin and Ray Connolly.

Hollywood stars Marilyn Monroe and Bruce Willis both stammered. UK celebrities who used to stammer or with stammers include Emily Blunt, Rowan Atkinson, Derek Nimmo and Gareth Gates.

MYTHS ABOUT STAMMERING

Myth 1: Children who stammer are not as intelligent as other children

Because we tend to associate intelligence with an ability to communicate, it is sometimes assumed that children who stammer are less intelligent than other children. There is exactly the same range of intelligence among children who stammer as there is among non-stammering children.

Myth 2: Parents are to blame for their child's stammer

This is a very persistent myth. Even in the film *The King's Speech*, the impression was given that the king may have developed a stammer because his parents were cold and unaffectionate. This notion has often been repeated in the media. No one would dream of suggesting that parents cause their children to be dyslexic or to be short-sighted. Parents do not cause stammering.

Myth 3: Stammering is caused by nerves

Because they speak hesitantly, it is often assumed that children may stammer because they are nervous. In books or on TV, children who stammer are often portrayed as nervous or lacking in confidence. In the *Harry Potter* books, and in many other books, there are references to characters 'stammering nervously'. Numerous studies have shown that people who stammer are no more nervous than the general population (Bloodstein and Ratner 2008). On the other hand, having a stammer may cause a child to be more nervous. Being nervous does not help anyone's fluency, but it is not the cause of stammering.

Myth 4: Stammering is caused by an event

Some children and their parents say they recall an event – a family row or the birth of a sibling – that happened around the time when the stammering began. However, such events occur in the lives of all children, and only a minority of children stammer. In some cases, an event may have been the trigger rather than the cause of the stammer in a child whose speech was already vulnerable. It is more likely that the timing was purely coincidental.

Myth 5: Children who stammer are shy and lack confidence

Because children who stammer may not speak in class or in groups, it is often assumed that they are shy and unconfident. But children have told us that while the reaction of other people can affect their confidence, they feel no different to anyone else. There is just as wide a range of personality types among children who stammer as there is among the general population.

Myth 6: People who stammer need help to speak

One of the things that can upset children who stammer is when people finish their sentences for them. People who stammer can appear to be very uncomfortable when trying to force out their words, but they tell us they really don't want other people who think they know what they are about to say to finish their sentences.

Myth 7: Stammering is 'catching'

Some parents have told us that they are afraid that because one of their children stammers, other children in the family may start to stammer too. Evidence is gathering that stammering has a genetic, physiological component to it, and it is highly unlikely that children would develop a stammer because they are copying the speech patterns of a sibling.

Myth 8: Stammering can be 'cured'

Parents often ask us if stammering can be cured. This makes it sound like some kind of illness – which it is not. There are courses and techniques that will help to reduce the stammer – it may even seem to disappear. However, many children find it exhausting to use techniques each time they speak and they may relapse. Many children learn to manage their stammer and to live with it. There is no 'cure' for stammering, but there is much that can be done to help.

Myth 9: Being left-handed causes stammering

In the 1930s and 1940s therapists believed that there might be a connection between having a stammer and being left-handed. An article called 'The Cure for Stammering' in an American magazine in 1940 stated that 'a young child stammers because he has been forced to change from a left-handed to a right-handed way of doing things' (DeWitt Miller 1940). In some societies where it is considered better to be right-handed it is believed that coercing naturally left-handed people to use their right hands may cause them to stammer. However, there is no connection between being left-handed and having a stammer.

Myth 10: Stammering is a deliberate act

Many people assume that because a child is capable of speaking fluently one day or in one situation, he must be able to speak fluently all the time. Teachers who have heard a child speaking fluently sometimes assume the stammer is attention-seeking behaviour or that the child is 'putting it on'. Stammering may fluctuate for a number of reasons, but not because a child is switching it on and off at will.

Chapter 2

HOW IT FEELS TO HAVE A STAMMER

WHAT CHILDREN SAY
'It's so frustrating'

> 'Sometimes I want to say something and I can't say a single word. The people around me don't even know that I'm trying to talk, that I'm trying to force out what I want to say and by the time I get it out they'll have already moved on. It's so frustrating.'
>
> *Joe, 15*

> 'I can't say what I want to say half the time – I get so angry at it. My talking makes me feel frustrated. It's a big personal challenge for me, and something that I have to overcome.'
>
> *Ibrahim, 13*

Imagine you're with a group of friends. The conversation is running along, people are cracking jokes, telling stories, having a laugh. Your mind is racing and you think of something really funny to say. There's a break in the conversation and you open your mouth to speak, then… nothing. Everyone is looking at you, there's an awkward silence and then someone else starts to talk. The thing you wanted to say goes unsaid. The interesting thought you had formed remains in your head. No one hears it. That's why people who stammer get so frustrated.

'You feel left out'

> 'Having a stammer is not a very good thing to have coz you don't join in on any activities that require speaking and you feel left out.'
>
> Wayne, 9

> 'People make me lonely because I can't get out what I want to say and they just ignore me. I feel lonely because no one is doing anything with me and people do stuff with people who are just normal. Sometimes I say to myself that I have no friends.'
>
> Thomas, 8

Children who stammer describe a vicious cycle. Because they're worried about stammering they opt out of activities… When they summon the confidence to take part they may be excluded, which further dents their confidence.

In some situations the listeners may not realise the person is trying to say something. Some types of stammering involve periods of silent 'blocking', and you can only tell that the child is trying to speak if you look closely at him or her. By the time the 'block' has passed, the conversation may have moved on and the child is left feeling frustrated and upset.

We're not used to waiting for several seconds for someone to speak. Some adults and children can react sensitively when they are aware of a stammer but groups of children at school have a tendency to talk over one another and interrupt. It can be a tough environment for a child who stammers.

'I'm the only one'

> 'Sometimes I feel like I'm the only one in the world who stammers.'
>
> Abed, 7

Stammering can be a lonely experience. Many children who stammer do not know anyone else who does. They may feel they have to hide their difficulty. Some will do anything to avoid speaking in front of others. Because of this their talent and ability can be overlooked.

The parents of children who stammer are often beside themselves with worry. A mother of a teenage girl told us recently: 'Everything she thinks about doing, her stammer just comes in the way of it. It makes her scared to do anything. It totally affects her whole life, I think it controls her life.'

'People think you're not very bright'

> 'People usually judge you by your first appearance and if the first thing you do is talk funny people think that you're not very bright or that you just aren't very clever.'
>
> Ahmed, 10

> 'Some people think that I'm dumb because I don't speak or answer anything. Some people actually think I'm not as intelligent as people who speak a bit more fluent than me.'
>
> Dylan, 8

Children who stammer say that people make assumptions about their intelligence. We associate intelligence with an ability to communicate, so children who always put up their hands to speak in class or who offer to read aloud or to do a presentation are generally seen as the bright ones.

As we have already stated, the range of intelligence among the population of people who stammer is just the same as it is among those who don't and many of the young people we have known who stammer are straight 'A' students.

'People laugh at me'

'When I feel upset it's because people laugh at me, so I feel upset, annoyed, frustrated, depressed.'

Abigail, 8

'Every time I want to ask a question I can't because I get scared of my stammer and then everybody around me starts to giggle and to snigger.'

Harry, 9

Children who stammer sometimes adopt physical ticks or mannerisms, which can look a bit strange to others. In their desperation to get their words out, they may blink repeatedly, put their head back or stick out their tongue. For a stammering child, the sight of their listeners pulling faces, sniggering, or exchanging knowing looks can be devastating.

We would never think it acceptable to laugh at someone who was physically disabled or blind, but the same doesn't seem to apply to stammering. Some children tell us they feel they have to laugh when they are being mocked, for fear of seeming not to have a sense of humour.

'You lose your confidence'

'My stammer was pretty horrible at times. I just wanted to say something like a good joke and I just couldn't and it was really demoralising. Once you start to feel bad and you lose your confidence, you start speaking less and say less than you want to and it gets worse and worse.'

David, 15

Those of us who don't stammer take for granted that we can give our names, say what we want to eat or drink, ask for a bus or train ticket or describe what we did that day.

For a child who stammers, the daily experience of struggling to articulate the most basic things and the drip-drip effect of being overlooked can do serious damage to his confidence. So, while nervousness is not a cause of stammering, having a stammer can most certainly cause a child to become nervous and less self-assured.

'You appear different to who you really are'

> 'Because I don't speak or say much, some people don't know what I'm thinking or what I'd like to say and they just think I'm that kid who's got a stammer.'
>
> Ahmed, 10

> 'If you have a stammer you are avoiding things you wouldn't avoid if you didn't have a stammer and you appear to be a different person to who you really are.'
>
> Max, 20

Children who stammer often say that their mouths are lagging way behind their thoughts. They might have a fantastic sense of humour and strong opinions, they might want to disagree with what has just been said, or answer back when someone makes a nasty quip. 'That kid who's got a stammer' might be the wittiest boy in the room. He just doesn't get a chance to show it.

This dislocation between a child's personality and the way that he is seen is very unsettling. It can be like being invisible. Having a stammer can diminish even the most upbeat young person's confidence.

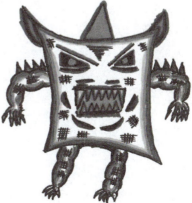

My stammer

'For me, it isn't that much of a problem'

> 'If I meet new people I try and tell them "Hi, I've got a stammer, don't worry about it, it's not bad, I'm not worried about it so you shouldn't either." And then once I've got that off my chest, everything's much easier. For me stammering isn't that much of a problem.'
>
> James, 16

> 'People do tend to think of me as different to everyone else coz I have a stammer but then everybody is different in their own way. People can make a big deal out of it but personally I just roll with it.'
>
> Eric, 15

Having a stammer affects different children in different ways. Some cope pretty well, while others really struggle and feel angry or upset a lot of the time. The severity of the stammer is not necessarily proportional to how badly the child is affected by it. What appears to be a mild stammer can have a major impact on a child's life. While others who stammer quite severely can be very resilient, they say they can just 'roll with it'.

Chapter 3

WHAT HELPS, WHAT DOESN'T

'I think it's hard for other people coz it puts them in an awkward situation. They don't know what to do because it's hard to help, and hard to know what to do.'

Emre, 14

Parents, friends and relatives of children who stammer want to do everything they can to help. But what may seem obvious – finishing off the sentence of the person who is stammering – can be the very thing they don't want us to do. We asked children and young people who attended the Michael Palin Centre to tell us what helps and what doesn't. This is what they told us…

WHAT MAKES IT WORSE
'Just hurry up!'

> 'The comments like "hurry up!" or "spit it out!" – people think they're being a bit jokey, but in a way, well, in a very big way, they're being quite horrible and it's some of the worst stuff that could happen to a person who stammers.'
>
> *Jonas, 13*

Telling someone with a stammer to hurry up is very counterproductive. If he tries to speak faster he is likely to stammer more and a vicious cycle sets in. The added pressure of being told to hurry will make him feel stressed, which can make the stammer worse still. When children are able to keep calm and take their time they are more likely to be able to express themselves freely.

'When I'm put on the spot'

> 'People do try and hurry me up especially if they want to go somewhere so they just try and make me speak quicker. It's worse when I'm put on the spot coz it makes it feel like everyone's watching me.'
>
> *Ibrahim, 13*

> 'When I'm on the bus and there's people standing behind me or in class if I've got to read and I know I'm gonna get stuck. And if I'm being asked a lot of questions it makes me feel more uncomfortable and that would lead to me stammering more.'
>
> *Ahmed, 10*

Many of us are not keen to be the centre of attention. If we have to speak at a wedding or give a presentation we can dread it for weeks or even months. When the day finally arrives we can find that our mouths dry up, we babble nervously and our jokes fall flat.

For some children who stammer, the prospect of speaking in front of a group of people can be terrifying. And the fact that they are very nervous can make the stammer worse. Their whole body becomes tense, their breathing is affected and the more they try to get their words out the more they get stuck.

People who stammer find themselves in the spotlight every single day in situations we take for granted, like buying a bus ticket or asking for a packet of crisps in a shop. People behind them in the queue might start to tut and fidget. 'What's going on? Why doesn't he say anything? We haven't got all day!'

There will always be difficult situations in which people who stammer simply have to speak. But when we are aware that someone has a stammer we can help to reduce the pressure on him by not forcing him to speak if he doesn't want to, and by giving him time to speak if he does.

'If someone finishes off your sentence'

'If someone finishes off your sentence, first it might not be what you're going to say, and it would be unfair on you because you're the one talking who wants to say that thing or make that point – it's well, very annoying.'

Harry, 9

'I think people in general who don't know about stammering will try and finish your sentences for you. They probably think that it helps, whereas the majority of people who stammer want to finish their own sentences.'

Omer, 12

When we ask children and young people what upsets them the most about how other people react to their stammer, 'people finishing off my sentences' comes top of the list. Understandably parents and friends are desperate to help if a child is struggling to get his words out but children who stammer generally don't find it helpful when other people speak for them.

Sometimes the listener doesn't realise that the child is trying to speak because there is no sound coming out. Or she might think that by completing the child's sentence she's putting him out of his misery.

A child who stammers wants you to wait until he has finished his own sentence no matter how long it takes. Other people finishing off his sentences can make the situation worse, especially if they get it wrong and he has to start all over again.

Very occasionally a child has told us that when he is really struggling, he doesn't mind if one of his parents helps him out with a word – as long as he is very sure that they know which word he is trying to say. However it is very important to ask your child if he wants you to do this. It is nearly always best to let the child get his own words out, no matter how long it takes. The more he opts out, the more he will feel he cannot speak for himself. The more he tries and succeeds, the more his confidence will grow.

'They think they know what I'm trying to say'

> 'Sometimes people see me stammering and they think they know what I'm trying to say. But if they get it wrong I have to start over again which is really, really frustrating. I think me and most people who stammer would just rather say it ourselves.'
>
> Abassi, 9

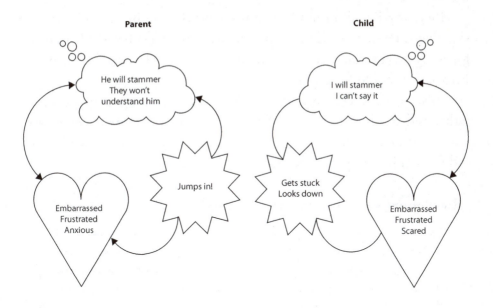

Parent   Child

He will stammer
They won't
understand him

I will stammer
I can't say it

Jumps in!   Gets stuck
                 Looks down

Embarrassed   Embarrassed
Frustrated   Frustrated
Anxious   Scared

A figure-of-eight cycle of negative feedback

To grow in confidence a child needs to speak in a variety of situations. The more he opts out, the more defeated he will feel. Parents naturally want to leap in and help out, but never being given the opportunity to speak in difficult situations will only increase the child's sense of defeat. He can come to believe that his parents have no confidence in his ability to speak for himself.

In discussions with groups of children and their parents at the Michael Palin Centre, we've identified a figure-of-eight cycle of negative feedback, as shown above.

Sam is in a restaurant with his parents. The waiter comes along and asks him what he would like to order. Silence. Sam thinks, 'Oh no! I'm going to stammer, I can't say "margarita pizza".' He becomes anxious, scared and embarrassed. He tries to say the word 'margarita' but he gets stuck and looks down.

Meanwhile his father thinks, 'He's going to stammer and the waiter won't understand what he's trying to say.' He feels embarrassed for Sam, for himself, for the waiter. He's worried and frustrated. So he jumps in: 'He'd like a margarita pizza please!'

There is relief all round but Sam knows that he just opted out. The experience reinforces his belief that he wouldn't have been able to order for himself. His confidence is dented a bit more. His dad feels bad too. Perhaps he should have waited…

This creates a feedback loop in which the feelings and actions of father and son fuel each other. Sometimes, when parents recognise this pattern, it helps them to stand back and let the child have a go himself rather than jumping in to rescue him each time.

'They ignore you while you're speaking'

'The worst thing people do to people with stammers is they ignore them when they're halfway through a sentence and they like ignore you while you're speaking – yeah, that's probably the worst thing they can do.'

Abassi, 9

'In some situations because of my stammering and coz I take quite a long time to say some things they'll just move on to the next person and ignore me. When people ignore me I feel upset quite a lot, upset and lonely.'

Harry, 9

It can be hard to listen if the child is taking longer to say something. There are often other things or people demanding our attention at the same time. It can be tempting to try to listen as we continue with other things, but this may be difficult for the child who stammers.

On the other hand, we cannot always stop what we are doing to give the child our undivided attention. This is unrealistic and unfair on the other children. It is about getting a balance. Sometimes parents will be able to listen carefully just when the child has something to say. Sometimes they need to say, 'I can't listen to you now, can we chat when this is done?' Sometimes the child who stammers will have to wait his turn while other children have their say.

We all like to be listened to, and when the child who stammers has his parent's full attention he will probably feel calmer and able to speak more fluently. He also needs to see that this has to fit in with the rest of the demands of family life.

'They treat you like a baby'

> 'Sometimes people say things they think are fine but I don't really like it. They ask me what my name is and if I take a long time to say it because I'm having trouble with my stammer, they say, "Have you forgotten it?" as a joke, but I might feel upset.'
>
> *Sean, 10*

> 'They spell things out to you and treat you like a baby because they don't know what a stutter is. I want them to care coz I don't like it if they don't care, I just go mad when they do that.'
>
> *Ahmed, 10*

Children and young people who stammer say they are often teased, and they frequently mention the fact that people who have other problems or disabilities are not teased in the same way. While it has become unacceptable to say to someone who has hearing difficulties, 'Oh, are you a bit deaf then?', children who stammer say they are sometimes asked something like, 'Don't you know your own name?'

People who stammer have sometimes been portrayed in sit-coms as comical characters, which may explain why some people still think it's OK to tease them.

Sometimes people think that when a child is stammering he has some kind of learning difficulty. With the best of intentions, they talk to him slowly and deliberately. This can be a frustrating and embarrassing misunderstanding for the child.

WHAT MAKES IT BETTER
'If I'm treated the same'

'People tend to put a label on anybody who has something slightly different to them. Stammering doesn't affect anything except what people hear. I'd like to be picked for football teams and stuff. I think I should be treated the same as any other people who have not got a stammer.'

Robert, 12

'Inside I know that we're all the same and just coz we've got something different about us doesn't mean we're not normal. It's just that some people take a bit longer to say what they want to say and if I'm treated the same I feel much better.'

Abassi, 9

Children and young people who stammer want to be given the same opportunities and choices as everyone else. They want to be invited to take part in school and social activities. They want to be considered for a part in the school play, the role of class representative, school prefect or councillor.

Parents and teachers sometimes assume that because a child has a speech impediment he won't want to join in activities that involve speaking. But some children find that they don't stammer when they are singing or acting so it's important they are given the chance to participate in activities that they'll enjoy and that will build their confidence. They may say no, but if they're asked at least they feel they've been treated equally and they've been given the same opportunities as their classmates.

People are often surprised to hear that young people sometimes tell us that there can be an advantage to stammering. For instance, if they have done something wrong, they may be let off lightly because of their stammer. Parents may notice that the child stammers more when he is in trouble, so they are more lenient with him. Teachers may treat children who stammer with kid gloves for fear of making the stammer worse.

While the young people clearly enjoy this unexpected benefit, there is a downside. It is not fair on other family members or school pupils if there are different rules for different children. It might also make it harder for the child to let go of the stammer if it is proving to be very useful to him.

'If people ignore my stammer'

> 'My friends all know me as me, but other people think of me as the boy who's got a stammer. I like it if people ignore my stammer and see me as I really am.'
>
> Harry, 9

> 'As a person I don't think that my stammer is my main characteristic really. I'm just a normal 15-year-old, but I have a speech impediment, and although it takes me longer to say things, it doesn't really stop me from saying the stuff that I want to say. It's just more of a time issue really.'
>
> Yousef, 15

It isn't always easy to ignore a stammer. But young people who stammer don't want the stammer to be their defining feature or characteristic. That's why speech and language therapists tend not to label people who stammer by calling them 'stammerers'.

In some ways it may be easier to overlook a physical disability. Once we have noted that a person is in a wheelchair we can concentrate on communicating with him or her as we would with an able-bodied person. But a stammer can act as a constant barrier to communication if we let it. That's why we need to learn how to listen to what a person who stammers is saying, rather than to focus on how they are saying it.

'Try to keep eye contact'

'Sometimes when the person is trying to get their words out no sound comes out but it's better if you wait for them, because they're trying to get out their words. Pay close attention to the person who stutters because it's usually through facial expressions that you can tell that they're trying to say something.'

Dan, 16

'Just try to keep eye contact with the person because if you look away they might think that you're getting frustrated and trying to speed this person up and that's probably the worst thing to do because the person starts to stammer. It's like a vicious cycle, so just stay calm and cool.'

David, 15

Some children take a while to get their words out and there can be long silences while they're trying to speak. It's important to maintain eye contact and to really listen to the child, rather than 'play act' that you are listening.

Children who stammer may become very sensitised to our response, and they can see from our facial expressions if we're bored, impatient or embarrassed. By concentrating on what the child who stammers is saying, rather than on his speech patterns, we can help him to feel he is successfully communicating with us. When he knows that we are listening he will feel more accepted and less pressurised.

'When you give me time to talk'

'If someone who stammers is having trouble speaking they should be given a bit more time because if everybody keeps interrupting then the person who has the stammer is gonna be thinking that there's no point in talking because they never get time to finish.'

Sean, 10

'My teacher gives me time. It makes me feel quite pleased. She gives me time to talk and give the answer and if I still don't get it she gives me some time to think it over and then she comes back to me again.'

Abigail, 8

Having to speak quickly usually leads to more stammering. Telling children to 'get on with it' only makes things worse. Subtler forms of pressure can also be applied – walking towards the door, looking away, glancing at a watch – all give a clear signal to the child who is stammering that you're too busy to listen, that he's taking too long and that you really have to get on.

By remaining calm, by listening closely and showing that you are happy to wait until he has finished what he wants to say, you will reduce any pressure the child is feeling to speed up and he will be more likely to speak fluently. Of course, as we have already said, this needs to be balanced with everything else that you are trying to do, and sometimes you will not be able to give your child a long and unhurried slice of your attention.

'Encourage me'

> 'People make me happier and more confident if they encourage me. They can encourage me by saying nice things, saying things that I can do, things that you are great at, nice things, any nice things.'
>
> *Sean, 10*

> 'It helps definitely, support and praise. The best thing a person can do is give me praise coz it gives me more confidence and then it's like I can do anything!'
>
> *Ahmed, 10*

Most of us like to receive praise when it is sincere and deserved. It lets us know that other people appreciate us and it helps to build our confidence, especially if we're not feeling good about ourselves.

Children who stammer may experience many knocks to their confidence and they are often extremely self-critical. They might judge their own performance harshly, tell themselves they're rubbish, and may believe everyone thinks they're stupid.

We can help to build a child's confidence by telling him what he's doing well and what his good qualities are. Sincerity is essential – children will see straight through 'sham' praise and instantly dismiss it. Praise expressed via a text message, a handwritten note or a school report is especially valuable as the child can re-read it whenever he likes.

'Just ask me how I feel'

> 'High pressure situations are difficult to deal with but people who stammer need some of them to get out of their comfort zone. I think only the child who stammers has the choice of whether they want to do it and at the end of the day they shouldn't be forced to do anything.'
>
> *Pete, 17*

'I think that if people could just ask me how I feel and how I want to be treated then they can take that into account and it could help to make me feel much happier.'

Harry, 9

Parents and teachers sometimes say that they're unsure about whether they should talk to a child about his stammer. If the subject is never raised, the child who stammers can feel he has a dark secret, that it's taboo or something to be ashamed of.

Young people say they would like parents, friends and teachers to ask them what they want us to do when they stammer. This alleviates tension around the stammer and gives the child the opportunity to tell us how he would like us to help and what he would like us to do when he's stammering.

There are no golden rules about how to help a child who stammers. He will have his own view on what is most helpful and this may change over time. An open dialogue will help both parties to feel more confident.

Chapter 4

PARENTS

HOW PARENTS MAY FEEL
'I felt isolated'

> I didn't know anybody else whose child had a stammer, so I felt isolated. We used to get quite distressed about it, not knowing what the future would hold for him.
>
> *Mother of 8-year-old boy*

Many children say they feel they are 'the only person in the world who stammers'. The parents of children who stammer can feel isolated too as they are unlikely to know other parents of children who stammer.

In groups at the Michael Palin Centre parents say that they derive great strength from one another, and that it's a relief to share their feelings with others who have had a similar experience. They are not judged when they admit to feelings of frustration or irritation. They laugh and sometimes cry together.

Parents of children who stammer often learn as much from other parents as they do from the therapists. The British Stammering Association and other self-help organisations also promote contact between parents.

'We're worried'

> He does control it but it's what's going on underneath that is the major problem for him. He's in bits inside. He gets very depressed about life. We're worried about how it's going to develop, about his

friendships, about relationships with other children, social skills, especially starting school.

Mother of 12-year-old boy

He always just takes himself off on his own. I worry a lot. As a mum you just want to do your best for him, you want for him to live a happy life, a full life. We want him to achieve his potential and do what he wants to do. People have actually walked away from him while he's talking. It breaks your heart.

Mother of 10-year-old boy

Parents worry about whether the child will make friends, how he'll manage at school, in oral exams, at interviews, about whether he'll get a job or get into college or university. Will he ever have a girlfriend, get married or have a family? The list goes on.

A common worry is that their child will be teased. Parents who also stammer (or used to stammer) may assume that their child will relive their own experiences, and parents who have been bullied themselves will be more fearful for their child.

Our work with parents is never going to eliminate their worries, but at the Michael Palin Centre we have found that the more parents know about stammering, and the more they can do to help, the less anxious they feel. We help parents to identify the things they already do to support their child's fluency and encourage them to continue doing them.

We make no rash promises that we can eliminate stammering, but we show parents how they can help their child to realise his potential in spite of his stammer.

'I feel for him'

You're trying to play a game or do homework with your child and you can't understand what he's saying, but you're aware that he's got so much to say and only a fraction of it comes out. I feel for him about the psychological distress because I think that's massive.

Father of 13-year-old boy

People who have little or no experience of stammering may not understand the level of distress it can create – in the person who stammers and in their parents.

To watch your child struggle day in and day out – not managing to say his name, opting out of conversations, being misunderstood – can be heartbreaking. Hard though it is at times, it's important to remember that even people with the most severe or entrenched stammers have overcome them or learned to live with them and have gone on to lead fulfilling and happy lives.

'I just can't help myself'

> I do get irritated with her. Especially after the therapy course when her speech was really nice. I'll say, 'Where are your shoes? I'm in a hurry! Where are they?' I know I shouldn't be doing that. I'll say, 'What time is it?' She'll go, 'Oh aaaaaah' and I'll say, 'Oh, let me have a look!' I just can't help myself.
>
> *Mother of 14-year-old girl*

> We have seen him being really fluent. But we get a glimpse of it and then it disappears. I've even said, 'They've taught you how to do this… why can't you do it?' It can lead to lots of frustration.
>
> *Mother of 10-year-old boy*

Parents can feel exasperated – with him, with themselves and with the whole situation. They don't want to get irritated but they can't help it. He's started to tell you what happened at school today, it's taking half an hour, and the bank's about to close.

Parents can feel perplexed if their child doesn't seem to be trying to overcome the stammer – particularly if they've spent a lot of time (and sometimes money) on speech and language therapy sessions in which he has learned techniques to help his fluency.

Slowing down your speech and running words together require enormous concentration and the effort can be exhausting. For that reason many children find it easier to stammer. While we want to give them all the tools they need to try to reduce the stammer, they need to feel that we accept them when they stammer too.

'You might have done something to cause it'

> Why didn't we deal with it before? What were we thinking? The thought that he may have been able to get rid of his stammer if only we'd acted earlier makes me feel very bad.
>
> *Mother of 13-year-old boy*

> You always worry that you might have done something to cause it. Maybe you interrupted him too much, talked over him, asked him too many questions. Getting therapy is good but when you find out what you can do to help, you realise you've done all the wrong things.
>
> *Mother of 9-year-old boy*

One of the common myths about stammering is that the child's parents may be to blame. Children who stammer live in all sorts of families with a whole range of parenting styles. Children who are brought up very harshly, who suffer deprivation or who experience all sorts of traumas do not go on to stammer.

There is now strong evidence that stammering is a result of genetic and physiological factors (see Chapter 1). At the Michael Palin Centre we give parents up-to-date information about stammering and we do everything to reassure them that they have not caused their children to stammer.

'We wrapped her in cotton wool'

> I worry about her not having any friends, about her not interacting, not finding a husband, all the nice things I've been able to do. I think the hardest thing is the feeling inside that this child of yours must feel lonely because of the stammer.
>
> *Mother of 13-year-old girl*

> We think we shouldn't have wrapped her up in cotton wool so much. We should have allowed her to practise talking more with people of her own age.
>
> *Mother of 14-year-old girl*

Throughout this book children and young people have made it clear that they want to speak for themselves, use their own words, finish their own sentences, lead their own lives.

Parents are often tempted to rescue their child if they see him floundering in front of other people. But treating him with kid gloves is unlikely to help him cope more easily with his stammer in future. The best thing you can do for your child is encourage him to speak in difficult situations – even if he stammers.

SUPPORTING YOUR CHILD AT HOME

'Supportive families are really helpful coz they just help you to release all of the pressure and tension that builds up if you start to stammer a lot and it is just really useful because they help put you at ease.'

Moishe, 14

It can be a tough world out there for young people who stammer. Every day can be an obstacle course, trying to get a word in with your mates, sticking up for yourself in the school playground or having to read aloud in class. There are things parents can do to try to help their children at school, which we describe in the following pages.

However, it makes life a bit easier for children who stammer if they feel they have the love and acceptance of their parents and if their home environment is supportive, a safe place where they can take their time to speak and be heard.

Talking about the stammer

You're never sure whether it's better to try to ignore it or talk to them about it and, if so, what to say. You don't want them to think that it's this huge thing that you're thinking about the whole time but, on the other hand, you don't want it to become something that can't be mentioned.

Father of 8-year-old boy

Parents often wonder whether they should speak to their child about his stammer. Some say by ignoring it they hope it might go away. Others say they don't want to make an issue of the stammer, or they don't want to upset or alarm their child even more.

A surprising number of older children and teenagers tell us that they have never talked about their stammer to their parents or to anyone else. There has been a well-intentioned 'conspiracy of silence'. They say this makes them feel they have a secret condition that is embarrassing and shameful. They feel they have to hide their stammer, that people find it unacceptable.

We encourage parents to acknowledge the stammer, just as they would any other problem their child may have. We suggest that with young children they can say things like, 'Oh, that was hard to say, wasn't it! Well done, you got there in the end.' Giving their speech problem a name may be helpful for the child, but take care to talk about the stammer rather than labelling the child as 'a stammerer'.

Ups and downs

> You can hardly notice it for a few months, then it comes back with a vengeance. Ups and downs the whole way, there's no real pattern to it. Sometimes you can't put your finger on what has kicked it off again. Sometimes he stammers even more when he's relaxed or on holiday because he doesn't have to try to perform for anyone. He lets go of it and stammers even more.
>
> *Father of 12-year-old boy*

Stammering can change from day to day, week to week, month to month. It can vary at different times of the day; it can seem mild at times and severe at others. Looking for signs that it is getting worse can make parents – and the whole family – more anxious.

On the other hand, constantly looking for improvement can be equally distressing when the improvement doesn't happen or is short-lived. If parents make too much of improvements in the child's speech, he (and they) will only feel worse if his speech deteriorates again.

Parents who stammer

Given the genetic nature of stammering, it's not unlikely that a child who stammers will have a parent with a stammer. That parent will understand what the child is going through. He or she will know what it feels like to stammer and the range of reactions the child is likely to encounter.

But the child's personality, his particular stammering behaviour and the way his friends react could all be very different. Parents who stammer can become over-protective and fuel their child's anxiety. For example, they may be afraid that their child will have no friends at school because they didn't have any.

A parent who stammers can provide a positive role model for the child by showing that it needn't be a barrier to a successful life. A child who can think 'having a stammer didn't hold my dad back' may benefit more from that than from years of therapy.

Parents who used to stammer are often less concerned. They're right to be optimistic as their child is more likely to grow out of it. However, if he has been stammering for some years, spontaneous recovery is less likely and therapy could help him to be a confident and competent communicator, even if he continues to stammer into adulthood.

Children with siblings

> When the others interrupt him we'll say, 'Be quiet! John's talking! Let him speak!' Then everyone has to wait for him to finish. Sometimes the others get fed up and wander off.
>
> *Mother of 9-year-old boy*

We say a lot in this book about the importance of listening, of good eye contact, and of waiting for the child to finish what he wants to say. But brothers and sisters also need to speak and be heard.

One parent told us recently, 'Whenever he is stammering, I feel I have to stop what I'm doing and give him my full attention.' There is a danger that parents may try so hard to allow the child who stammers to speak that the other children in the family feel left out or ignored.

When children come to the Michael Palin Centre for therapy, we invite their siblings to join in for one session. One of the reasons for this is because siblings can feel left out while both parents attend therapy with the child who stammers. They can feel that the child who stammers is special, while they are not.

It's tempting to take a softer line with the child who stammers – especially if he stammers more when he is in trouble. But remember that he is capable of using his stammer to get out of doing things he doesn't want to do. Treat him exactly the same way as you would any other child. Rules should apply to all – you don't get let off doing the washing-up just because you stammer.

The only child

> We sit there at mealtimes and it can take him so long to answer a question, all the attention is on him. We're sitting quietly waiting and watching, but the dinner's getting cold and everyone feels really stressed.
>
> *Mother of 9-year-old boy*

A single child will often receive his parents' full attention. While this can be great for him in one way – his parents have more time to spend with him and they can concentrate fully on his needs – there is a downside.

Sometimes there aren't other distractions and the only child who stammers may feel the focus of all the attention. He may pick up on any anxiety his parents are feeling. Try to be aware of this and think of ways of relieving any pressure on the child. Take turns to spend time with him and try to make mealtimes light and easy. Be aware that conversation between adults may be more sophisticated and quite a challenge for a child to join in.

In social situations

> I realise that I do too much for him. I talk for him, I do everything for him, and it's going to be a matter of being cruel to be kind. He's going to have to start talking more, talk to different people, ask for things. I have to keep reminding myself – it's his stammer, it's not mine. It's his life, he can try to do something about it. I have to try to accept that. I have to accept him for who he is really.
>
> *Mother of 11-year-old boy*

Some young people say they find talking to new people hard, especially adults or relatives. Tricky situations include having to talk in the car or at after-school clubs, getting a bus or train ticket, buying something in a shop and talking at parent-teacher events.

Parents feel very torn – should they step in and help or let the child struggle on? Jumping in gives the child the message that you don't think he can manage. You may assume he can't cope when he feels fine about speaking. Also, if you constantly rescue him he will never be able to practise in difficult situations. Even if he stammers, the fact that he tried will help build his confidence.

You can ask your child if, and how, he'd like you to support him in social situations. Together you can decide that next time he's in a restaurant he'll order for himself while you silently support him. He'll see that you have confidence in him. It doesn't matter if he stammers – give him praise for trying. It's about being brave and a bit more independent.

Parents of teenagers often tell us that they have recently become more withdrawn. This is pretty common among teenagers, whether they stammer or not. However, parents should be alert to sudden changes in behaviour which could indicate that something is wrong. Talking to your child, the school, your child's friends, their parents or a GP may help you decide what to do.

If there is more than one language

Using more than one language does not cause stammering, so it is fine to use two languages at home. Learning a second language will be an enormous asset to your child, especially if this is the language spoken by the wider family.

Children who speak more than one language may stammer equally in both, or more in one than the other. Sometimes they stammer more in the language that they find easier because they are speaking more quickly.

The most important thing for a child who is learning to speak is that he hears a rich language model. Switching between languages is not a problem.

It's important to focus on helping your child feel he is communicating with you successfully. Continue speaking your chosen language/s to your child even if he replies to you in a different language.

The following websites offer information about using more than one language at home:

www.londonsigbilingualism.co.uk

www.speechtherapy.co.uk

www.bilingualism.co.uk

www.stammering.org/bilingual.html

www.stutteringhelp.org.

ADVICE AND SUGGESTIONS

In this section we suggest some ways that you can build your child's confidence and help him to become more fluent. These suggestions won't work for everyone. If you try one out and it isn't working or it doesn't feel right for you and your child, just drop it and try something else.

Praise him

Comment on your child's strengths and good qualities. He may be kind and patient with younger children, he may be brave, thoughtful or helpful at home. He may be talented at football, playing a musical instrument or drama.

If praise is specific and descriptive he will be less likely to brush it off or disregard it and it will help him develop a positive self-image. So, rather than 'Great!', 'Brilliant!' or 'Well done!' it's better to say, 'That drawing looks exactly like our dog – you are very artistic,' or 'You've really managed to master that tune on the piano perfectly – you are very tenacious.' Your child can't argue with the facts of what you have described and the label 'artistic' says something about him as a person. Praising your child in this way just once a day will really boost his confidence.

Take turns to talk

When we are in a group, we often overlap or interrupt each other. This is completely normal social behaviour. But it can be harder for a child who stammers if he is rushing to finish what he wants to say before someone else butts in or if he is rushing to interrupt someone else. You could help your child by ensuring that everybody in the family listens to each other and nobody interrupts the speaker. He will then feel able to take his time and this can help him to be more fluent. It's also important to remember to keep things fair – other family members should have their say as well as the child who stammers.

At the Michael Palin Centre we teach families 'The Microphone Game'. We sit in a circle with the microphone in the middle (a wooden spoon will do). Only the person who has the microphone is allowed to talk and everyone is to have a turn. We might start with 'My favourite food is…' When the first person has finished, he replaces the microphone and someone else takes over. This goes on until each person has had a few turns.

With older children we play 'Build a Story'. The first person with the microphone begins 'One dark night, a strange light appeared in the middle of an empty field…' Whoever wants to continue this story picks up the microphone. It's better to do this randomly rather than working around the circle. Watching the microphone coming round the circle towards them might be very stressful for some children.

The rules are:

- only the person with the microphone is allowed to talk

- everybody should get a turn

- we listen to each other

- interrupting is not allowed

- it should be fair – nobody should get a longer turn.

Slow down

Many of us have a fast pace of life and it isn't always easy to slow things down, but perhaps there are ways of reducing the pressure, or creating a quiet time in the day when a child has time to gather his thoughts and speak without feeling rushed.

Routine

A surprising number of parents tell us that their child's fluency is usually better when he is in his usual routine. Maybe the predictability of life makes him feel more in control, which helps him to feel calmer. Regular meals and sufficient sleep seem to be important. Parents and children often say that the stammering is worse when they are tired.

There are certain times when our normal routines are disrupted, which can be a great relief to parents but may have a detrimental effect on the child who stammers. Holidays, either at home or away, can be times when the child unexpectedly starts to stammer more. Maybe it is because of the lack of routine, the unfamiliar environment, the late nights. We are not suggesting that families do not go on holiday but it may be worth thinking about how you can keep your child on an even keel at this time.

Another time that parents often report a dip in fluency is during major religious and public holidays. The combination of excitement, late nights, staying guests, unusual mealtimes and, sometimes illness may be the reason for the increase in stammering. It may be helpful to look out for signs that your child is starting to struggle and make a few small changes to help him to cope with the disruption to normal life.

Be consistent

Sometimes parents don't see eye to eye about how to deal with their child who stammers. It's important to reach agreement on the best approach. Having conflicting approaches is unhelpful and confusing for the child. There's enough stress to go around without parental squabbling.

Sometimes one parent will notice that the other is doing something unhelpful, like interrupting or firing too many questions at him when he gets in from school. It's better to talk about this out of earshot of the child. And make sure one parent doesn't take all the criticism. Try to reduce the pressure on one another, as well as on the child who stammers.

One-to-one time

Most of us like to receive – and give – some undivided attention. It can really help the child to have a bit of one-to-one time when neither you nor your child has to think about anything else and you can just focus on each other. Just five minutes will help. In a busy family lifestyle, you may find it useful to have a brief, regular slot with each child.

During one-to-one sessions you can try out some of the ways of helping his fluency that are suggested below. Don't introduce them all at once – select one or two and see how it goes. None of them will work straight away, so gradually incorporate the helpful ones, ditching the ones that are not.

LISTEN TO WHAT HE'S SAYING, NOT HOW HE SAYS IT

When a child is stammering, try not to focus on how he is talking. Concentrate on what he is saying. If he stammers, act as if he is being fluent, maintain eye contact and wait until he has finished speaking.

PAUSE – THEN GO AT HIS SPEED

Most adults speak more quickly than their children. A child who stammers needs time to think and plan what he wants to say and he may need extra time to co-ordinate the muscles involved in speaking. You can slow down the pace by introducing a little pause before you speak. It can also help to try to match your child's speed of talking.

It's usually unhelpful to tell the child to slow down. Adults find it hard enough to change their own speed so we shouldn't ask children to do it. He may be able to slow down for a moment or two, but it's unlikely to last – and you'll both end up feeling frustrated. It may be better to say 'Take as much time as you like…there's no hurry.'

LET HIM FINISH

If the child is really struggling, it can be tempting for parents to finish his sentence. But children who stammer tell us they don't like this. They don't want us to guess, they would rather we hear them out. Very occasionally a child will tell us that he doesn't mind when his parents help him out with a word here and there if he's pretty sure they know what he's trying to say. But it's important to check that the child is happy for you to do this. Just ask him what he wants you to do when he gets stuck.

USE QUESTIONS CAREFULLY

When a child is asked a question, he is put on the spot to respond. His ability to answer fluently will depend on how difficult the question is and how good his language skills are. You could help your child to answer more fluently if you:

- avoid complicated questions

- give him lots of time to reply

- let him answer the first question before asking another

- turn questions into statements that allow him to speak if he wants to, e.g. 'I bet you enjoyed art today.'

SUPPORTING YOUR CHILD AT SCHOOL
At primary school

'Well, I'd like my teachers and my school to know what causes stammering and what emotions I feel when I'm stammering and just what stammering means to people. I haven't told my teacher about it because I'm too scared and I think it would make me feel better if I did.'

Freddie, 9

'I do think that teachers can help because they sometimes let me have a bit more time on one of those days when I'm stammering more. Also the teachers told me that if there's a day when I don't feel like saying anything then I don't have to, and if I want to then I can, so they're giving me the choice, they're not saying I have to.'

Philip, 10

Most parents worry when their child first goes to school or when he changes school. Parents of children who stammer may have extra concerns. They worry that the child will be bullied or laughed at by other children. They worry that he won't speak in class and that the teacher won't know about stammering or how to handle it.

On the other hand, they don't want to make a big fuss because they know he has to learn to fend for himself. They also want him to be treated normally, like all the others in his class. It's hard to get the balance right.

The first thing to do is to inform your child's school about his stammer. His class teacher is usually the best person to tell. Sometimes parents feel the teacher is not very sympathetic or interested, so it is better to get in touch with the school's special needs coordinator (SENCO) or the head teacher.

It's important to explain that your child may struggle in different situations at school – asking for lunch, speaking to the school secretary or caretaker, talking in the playground. Ask for all the staff who will come into contact with your child – lunchtime supervisors, office staff, teaching assistants, playground attendants – to be made aware of the stammer.

Some everyday activities in school can be tricky for a child who stammers – like being asked to say his name during registration. There are ways of dealing with this which don't impact on the other children, but which make a huge difference to the stammering child. We include a number of suggestions in Chapter 5.

Stammering Information Programme

'There are some teachers who always get it right and there are some who are too hard, and a few who are patronising.'

Rory, 16

Parents can tell their child's school about the Stammering Information Programme, which has been produced by the Michael Palin Centre to educate school staff about stammering. In the programme, which comprises a DVD and downloadable advice sheets, children who stammer talk about their experiences at school, and describe what helps and what doesn't.

The Programme, which is free of charge, is available on the Michael Palin Centre website www.stammeringcentre.org/guides.

At secondary school

> Secondary school seemed like such a big jump. It felt like we were throwing him to the lions.
>
> *Father of 12-year-old boy*

'At secondary school there's an atmosphere of competitiveness and to be the coolest you have to be the loudest, most confident, and also, kids at that age are cruel. Using your voice becomes much more important.'

Max, 20

It can be harder for parents to support their son or daughter at secondary school. Typically, the school is much larger and he will have fleeting contact with his form tutor. Students move around the school and see a number of different teachers.

The form tutor may be the first point of contact. It's important to ask how all the teachers he will have that year can be made aware of his stammer. The SENCO may also be able to help as may the head of year, head of house or a pastoral head.

If your son is encountering problems there may be a school counsellor or school mentor he could talk to. Whatever the system, try to make sure that all the staff who come into contact with him are told about his stammer in advance and are given some guidance.

SUBJECT CHOICES

A student who stammers may be influenced by his speech when it comes to choosing subject options. It's possible that he will opt for subjects that don't involve speaking or oral presentations.

Of course he may genuinely prefer the subjects he has chosen but if you think he may be missing out on subjects that interest him and that he's good at because of his fear of oral work, then you could discuss this with him.

If he says he would like to study French but couldn't bear to read aloud, you could ask for a meeting with the French teacher to explore the possibilities. He may be able to do oral presentations in front of one teacher or in a small group and the teacher could inform the exam board that his oral work will be affected by his stammer.

If he's being bullied

'I'm the only one in school with a stammer and I feel like the odd one out. I've been bullied at school and that makes me sad and angry. I feel scared and nervous most of the time.'

Francesca, 9

Just because a child has a stammer doesn't mean he will be bullied at school. But sadly, many of the children we see at the centre say they have been teased or bullied. Parents should be aware of this and regularly check in with the child about how the other pupils are reacting. Changes in the child's behaviour may flag up a problem at school. Children often don't tell anyone that they are being bullied for fear that complaining will make the bullying worse.

If you suspect something is amiss, or if your child seems moody or depressed, explore it with him gently. It may help to talk to his friends or their parents. You could also tell your child's teacher or form tutor that although he hasn't reported any bullying, you are worried that something might be wrong.

If your child has told you that he is being bullied you should decide the best course of action together. Some parents encourage their children to stick up for themselves even to the point of hitting back at the bully. But if your child reacts violently he may end up getting into more trouble than the bully.

Here are some strategies children have used:

IGNORE THE BULLY AND WALK AWAY

> 'I had a bully in primary school and it put my confidence back really bad. I was bullied a bit in senior school, but if you ignore them and stick up for yourself they just get bored.'
>
> Hamid, 15

Most bullies are looking for a reaction and if the victim shows that he's upset or angry the bullying has been successful. If the child can hide his feelings and walk away, the bully isn't getting the desired result and the bullying might stop.

SAY YOU HAVE A STAMMER

> 'People don't really take the mick any more but when I was in primary school I remember that someone was making fun of me. I wasn't quite sure what to do then, but if asked how come I talk like this now, I find it better to tell them because when they know about it they know how to deal with it.'
>
> Stephen, 16

Many children think this is a bad idea until they see the effect when they try it out in role play. We ask the child to say something to the therapist or the parent, such as 'Your ears stick out!' (with the adult having suggested what they would be prepared to be 'teased' about). The 'victim' then says, 'I know they do – they have always been like that.' It is interesting to see how this often takes the wind out of the sails of the 'bully'. Children often realise that it can be very disarming just to say, 'I know I stammer. My words get stuck and I can't get them out.'

TELL A TEACHER

'If in class a person is stammering and someone laughs at them they should be told off coz if someone was in a wheelchair and you laughed at them just coz they couldn't walk it would be a serious matter.'

Sean, 10

We encourage children to tell teachers if they are being bullied. Most schools have anti-bullying policies, although this doesn't necessarily eliminate bullying. The child may need his parents' support in reporting the bullying. Some schools have anonymous reporting systems or 'peer mentors' to try to tackle bullying. Even if your child doesn't think it will make a difference, try to encourage him to report the incident so that it is at least recorded.

ASK FRIENDS TO SUPPORT YOU

'My friends give me support and it makes me feel quite happy coz then it's like they're all standing behind me and they want me to do well and they want me to get rid of my stammer.'

Harry, 9

Bullying is more likely to happen when a child is on his own and good friends won't mind if they're asked to support a child who feels vulnerable or who is being bullied. The support of his friends can make a child feel more confident and it may also help to deter the bully if he thinks he's taking on a group rather than one vulnerable person.

GETTING HELP WITH BULLYING

There are a number of organisations to help children who are being bullied and their parents:

Beatbullying

Details at www.beatbullying.org.

The British Stammering Association

Details at www.stammering.org.

Bullying UK

Details at www.bullying.co.uk.

ChildLine

Details at www.childline.org.uk.

Chapter 5

TEACHERS

'My teachers could help me if they knew how it affects my life. Because if all the teachers actually understand the stutter then they'll be able to deal with it properly, so the student can get an opportunity to say what he wants to say.'

Ahmed, 10

Children spend a significant part of their lives at school. What happens at school – whether you have friends, whether you feel included, whether you feel liked, respected or listened to – can affect the rest of your life.

At the Michael Palin Centre we have learned that the way teachers respond to children who stammer can make a big difference to the way they feel about themselves. Over the years, hundreds of children have attended the centre to get help with their stammering. They invariably talked about their school experiences and it is very clear that a helpful and sensitive response from a teacher can have a positive impact on a child. Sadly, some children have told us that their confidence has been eroded by the way they were treated at school.

We think the best way for teachers to learn how they can help and support children who stammer is to listen to the children themselves.

WHAT CHILDREN SAY ABOUT SCHOOL
'I try to avoid questions'

'Well, sometimes I give short answers so I don't have to say as much so I don't stammer in front of people. I try to avoid questions. The worst thing a teacher can do to me is make me stand up and read something in front of a crowd of strangers I don't know so I stammer a lot and they all laugh at me.'

Abigail, 8

'If a teacher said "I'll come back to you," I'll get a lot of tension in my stomach coz I realise that I'm going to be put on the spot and everyone's attention will be on me.'

Frankie, 12

Many young people say the hardest thing is being put on the spot or being forced to answer a question. It's hard for the teacher to know how to include a child who stammers in class activities without putting him under too much pressure.

We suggest that the teacher has a quiet word with the child to ask him what he'd like the teacher to do. Very often the child will come up with a good solution. Most children know that they need to practise speaking and they want to be given an opportunity to do so. They just don't want to be forced to speak when they're struggling to get their words out.

'They're not actually listening'

'Some teachers listen to you but not all the teachers. Some teachers pretend that they're listening but they're not actually listening, they're focusing on something else. Other teachers listen to what you have to say and respond to it.'

Carole, 15

We usually look at people when we are listening to them, but if the person is stammering we may feel uncomfortable and look away. This may be because we feel embarrassed for ourselves or for the person who is stammering, or we don't want to appear to stare – but looking away can give an unintended message.

A child may think that the teacher is feeling annoyed or impatient. He may think that the teacher has lost interest in what he has to say. These misunderstandings could crush a child's confidence in front of the rest of the class.

Maintaining natural eye contact, rather than a fixed stare, tells the child that you are listening, that you want to hear what he has to say and you are willing to wait.

We need to acknowledge that classrooms are busy places and a teacher cannot give each child unlimited, undivided attention. If a child who stammers approaches you at a busy time it is better to tell the child (who stammers) that you cannot listen to him at that moment, but you will come back to him, rather than pretend to listen when you cannot. It is then important to remember later to ask him what it was he wanted to say.

'They might not have the patience'

'The worst thing that a teacher's done to me is ignore you coz when you're stammering and they might not have the patience so they just ignore you and go deal with something else instead of listen to what you have to say.'

Andreas, 10

One boy said about his stammer, 'It feels like your brain is thinking at a higher level than your mouth is.' That's why it is so frustrating for children who stammer if people interrupt them, talk over them, or simply ignore them and start talking to someone else. They have interesting things to say, they just can't get their words out.

The mother of a boy who is an expert on dinosaurs told us, 'He's so intelligent but he hasn't got the tools to really tell people what he's thinking. When you do have a conversation with him it blows you away.'

If a child is struggling to speak it may be tempting to move on to another child rather than wait for him to finish. This can give a negative message to the child and to the rest of the class. The child who stammers may think that the teacher is annoyed with him or that what he was trying to say was wrong. To the class it sends a signal that you can ignore the child who is stammering.

'If I was given the time to think'

'After I've been asked a question if I was given the time to think about the answer it would be very helpful. If I was being asked lots of questions at once it would make me feel more uncomfortable and then that would normally lead to me stammering more. A good teacher doesn't interrupt what I'm saying, they give me time to speak and they also don't try and put pressure on me while speaking.'

Mathew, 12

'One of the worst things a teacher has done is to put their hand up and tell me to stop and think about my answer and they'll come back to me, and that really annoys me because I feel teachers should always be patient.'

Duncan, 9

Research into stammering has shown that many children who stammer have excellent language skills. If they are given more time to formulate what they are trying to say they may be more fluent. Therapy often involves helping the child to pause before he speaks and to speak more slowly, allowing the thoughts, sounds, words and sentences to flow.

Those of us who don't stammer don't usually rehearse what we are going to say before we speak. A child who stammers is sometimes told, 'Think before you speak' or 'Think about what you want to say, then say it.' These instructions may not be helpful. It would be better to give the impression that he can take his time, or to say, 'Don't worry, there's plenty of time.'

'My confidence goes down'

> 'When a teacher hasn't given me any praise so then my confidence goes down so I stammer a lot more.'
>
> Peter, 8

Stammering can create a vicious cycle. It can affect a child's confidence, which in turn leads to more stammering.

Encouraging the child to do the things that he enjoys and is good at will build his self-esteem. It also helps to praise and reward personal qualities such as being helpful, kind to others, reliable or truthful. Praising the child for these attributes, on his own, in front of other pupils or to his parents will boost his confidence.

Children who stammer may judge their fluency as an indicator of how well they are doing generally. It's important that they feel good about themselves despite their stammer. So it's best to focus on the fact that they tried to do something, not whether or not they were fluent. Teachers can help children by praising them for the effort they made, for the courage they showed or for the interesting things they said. They can also comment on good listening and communication skills.

'Sometimes it's good...sometimes it's bad'

> 'Well, sometimes it's good if I stand up and read, because I can practise my reading, but sometimes it's bad and I might stammer a lot.'
>
> Harry, 9

Most speech problems are pretty constant. One of the unusual things about stammering is that it can change quite dramatically from one day to the next. This can be baffling for teachers. Some children say their teachers have told them to stop stammering. The teachers think they are putting the stammer on because they have heard the children speaking fluently.

We still don't fully understand why stammers vary so much. We know that being excited, anxious or upset can make the stammer worse. Some children stammer more when they're tired or unwell, if they're trying to explain something complicated or if people are competing to speak. Trying to speak quickly usually makes it worse. Being angry affects children differently – some become very fluent while others can't utter a word.

A child who stammers is likely to have good and bad days at school. On bad days he may want to opt out of speaking in class, and on a good day he may want to read or take part in a drama lesson.

ADVICE AND SUGGESTIONS

We have interviewed many children and young people who have come to the Michael Palin Centre for therapy. We wanted to find out what they would like teachers to do to support them so that they could feel less stressed about their speech and fulfil their potential at school. Here are some of the things that they said:

Talk to the pupil

> 'I think the teacher has to speak to the pupil as soon as possible to find out what he'd like, how he wants them to respond, how often he wants the staff to ask them questions or ask them to read, and also do it regularly because people change how they feel about their stammer. One week might be quite good but another week might be quite bad.'
>
> *David, 15*

> 'If I had to advise a teacher then I would start off by just asking that child and their parents to come into school and have a conversation with them and ask them questions like whether they have any problems in certain situations, or if that child feels uncomfortable, for example if they have to say their name or read aloud.'
>
> *Carole, 15*

Teachers can find out how to support the child who stammers by asking him what would help, preferably when other classmates are out of earshot and when they have plenty of time to talk. Some children say they'd like the teacher to have a quiet chat with them on their own after class. Others would prefer their parents to be there.

The teacher could open the conversation with, 'I've noticed that you sometimes have trouble when you talk,' and then ask questions, such as:

- When you're finding it hard to speak, is there anything I can do, or should I just listen and let you finish?

- Would you like to put your hand up if you want to answer a question or read aloud?

- Is there anything we do in class that makes things more difficult for you?

- How can we make that less difficult?

- Is there anything you really like doing that you would like to do more of?

- Are any of the children in school giving you a hard time because of your speech?

- Would it help if you told me when you're having a difficult day?

- Would you like the class to know about your speech or is it better if we don't say anything?

- Would you like to tell them yourself, or would you like me to tell them?

These questions don't include the word 'stammer' or 'stutter' because the child may not use them to describe his speech.

Telling the class

> 'Well it would help if everybody knew that I stammered because they'll know I've not finished my sentence because I'm stopping to take a breath. If a teacher explains it then people will know what stammering is like and how it affects people's lives.'
>
> Abigail, 8

This is a tricky one for teachers. Some children say they think it would be better if their classmates knew they had a stammer. Others fear that things might get even tougher if everyone knew about the stammer.

Speech and language therapy often focuses on supporting the child to be more open. We encourage children to take small steps, starting with telling close friends or relatives about the stammer and building up from there. It clearly takes a lot of courage for a child to tell his classmates that he stammers, or to ask the teacher to tell them.

We would suggest that teachers take a lead from the child. If the child wants the class to be told, he should be asked whether he would like to be present. If he is happy to be there he may even be willing to answer their questions. This would demonstrate great courage and self-confidence.

Taking the register

> 'If the teacher is taking the register and if you have a stammer and you take longer to answer they might tell you off for not answering because they might not hear you. Because the register's important, the person who stammers might get upset about it coz they're trying to do their best.'
>
> Ibrahim, 13

'In my primary school was when I had most trouble with my stammer. It was with the register. The teacher said my name and I was trying to say it, and then she said my name again, thinking that I didn't answer, and I felt upset because I was answering – I was just taking a longer time.'

Alfie, 11

Answering the register can be a nightmare for some children who stammer. Whether the teacher goes round the room or reads out names in alphabetical order, the anticipation and the tension builds as the list of names goes on.

Rather than putting a child who stammers through this daily nightmare, the teacher could simply ask the children to either respond with a 'yes' or raise their hand when their name is called out.

Here are some other things that primary school teachers have tried with younger children:

- Read the names in pairs and have the children answer in pairs (children rarely stammer when they are speaking in unison with somebody else).

- Have all the children sing their responses (stammering normally disappears when a child sings or 'raps').

- Have the children clap on each syllable when they respond (speaking on a beat usually eliminates stammering).

- Vary the order so that the child who stammers is not first but neither does he have to wait too long before it is his turn.

Reading aloud

When he started secondary school and he had to read in English he dissolved in tears. They were going round the class, and he became very emotional. He tried, but when he cried the teacher took him out of the class and was very sympathetic. Since then he hasn't put him on the spot. Once or twice, at his own request, when he feels confident enough, he will volunteer.

Mother of 13-year-old boy

'If teachers used to ask me to read stuff in class I'd always become really hot and flustered and like "Oh no, what do I do now, what do I do!" I used to struggle through and I always noticed that the teachers used to give me shorter things to read and that was nice of them because it slowly helped to build my confidence.'

Harry, 9

Not all children who stammer want to opt out of reading aloud. Even those who stammer severely want to be given the choice.

One teenage boy told his mother that although he didn't like reading aloud in front of his class in English lessons, his teacher encouraged him to try, and once he had done it a few times, he was glad he'd done it. He said that reading aloud from time to time had helped build his confidence.

However, reading out loud can be difficult, even for skilled readers with excellent comprehension. Having a fixed text can put extra pressure on the child, especially if he uses 'starter' words or sounds, or if he changes words he finds hard to pronounce. The politician Ed Balls says he struggles with words beginning with the letter 'h' so he always rewrites scripts for speeches. His worst nightmare is having to read the Bible aloud as he cannot change it!

'Because when you read in class and you've got a stammer you feel a lot of pressure because everyone's waiting for you, it's silent, it's just your voice, and it's quite intense sometimes.'

Abassi, 9

'Reading around the room' can present extra pressures as the tension rises for the child who stammers. Selecting random children to read creates less pressure and the teacher can include the child who stammers if he wants to read.

Reading in small groups of three or four can be less stressful for a child who stammers. Longer multi-syllabic words are often more difficult to read aloud and the child may stammer more. Teachers can choose slightly shorter passages for children who stammer.

Stammering does not usually happen when children read in unison. They can be asked to read in pairs or in a group, or the teacher can read quietly with the child who stammers.

Answering questions

'If my teacher picked me to stand up and answer a question I'd feel like the teacher hadn't been paying attention because it's obvious that I have a stammer. But if I put up my hand then they'd know I want to speak.'

Charlotte, 14

A child who stammers will often prefer to volunteer to speak or answer a question by putting up his hand rather than being randomly chosen by the teacher. If he's having a difficult day with his speech he can opt out.

One child set up an ingenious system of communicating with his teacher: he would put his hand up with his fist closed to show that he knew the answer but didn't want to speak and he opened his hand if he was ready to say the answer in front of the whole class. By doing this he was able to participate more fully in the class, but he had more control over how much he spoke.

Assemblies and school plays

'If I was asked to stand in front of an assembly I would feel uncomfortable. But sometimes I stammer when we practise and on the actual day I can do it without stammering.'

Katrina, 14

Some people who stammer find that when they act, sing or adopt an accent, the stammer either disappears or they become more fluent. A number of famous actors have a history of stammering or still stammer. For example, the actor Emily Blunt said that drama helped her to overcome her stammer.

While some children who stammer like to perform, others hate it. But it shouldn't be assumed that a child who stammers will only ever want a backstage role in the school play. He should be asked if he'd like to take part – he may be a future star of stage or screen.

Teasing and bullying

'To all of the teachers, if you ever see anybody stammering and someone laughs it isn't very nice because the children are affecting the person who stammers. They're trying to make him have a bad life, so he stammers even more. I don't want that and nor do any of the other children who stammer. I would say to teachers – help us, and tell the other children to stop teasing us.'

Ahmed, 10

'I find it quite upsetting when I stammer in front of people that tease me. Some people go, "Is it a disability or is it contagious?" If they laugh at the person stammering, that should be taken as a serious offence coz if somebody was in a wheelchair and you laughed at them, it would be a serious matter.'

Denis, 16

Children who stammer are sometimes teased or bullied. Bullying can be very subtle and can go unnoticed by school staff. When a child who stammers is reading aloud, his classmates may only exchange a knowing look for him to feel humiliated.

Speech and language therapists encourage children to tell their teachers if they are being teased but they can find this very hard. Teachers can create a safe forum and an open dialogue, so that children can be honest about any problems they are having and they know they will be believed.

Circle Time or Citizenship lessons help to increase tolerance and we know of courageous children who have used these occasions to talk to their classmates about stammering.

On very rare occasions, children who stammer tell us that they have been mimicked or teased by a teacher. This gives a clear message to the other pupils that such behaviour is acceptable and puts the child in an impossible situation. We realise that such teachers are in a very small minority, but it seems important to make it known that this has been the terrible experience of a few children.

Presentations and oral exams

'My English teacher lets me do my oral tasks at lunchtime so then I am on my own, so I can just feel secure. I can be happier and I can still have my work finished.'

Alan, 14

There is currently a big emphasis on children doing verbal presentations to their peers and teachers. These can be a real challenge for the child who stammers. Teachers can help by discussing with the child whether he feels able to do this and what might be the best way to approach it.

There are a number of options. The child could do a joint presentation with one or two other students, with a slightly shorter contribution. He could make the presentation to a small group, or the teacher and one or two other students. If he really feels unable to present, he could contribute to the content of the presentation without having to read it out to the rest of the class.

Oral exams that form a part of learning a foreign language may also be something of an ordeal. It may help if the examiner is aware that the child stammers and may need more time.

Teachers often apply for special consideration or adaptation of the oral exam for children who stammer. This may involve allowing extra time. A speech and language therapist can support the child by sending a letter to request this.

RESOURCES FOR TEACHERS

The Michael Palin Centre

The 'Stammering Information Programme', which the centre has produced to educate school staff about stammering, comprises downloadable advice sheets and a DVD in which children who stammer talk about their experiences at school, and describe what helps and what doesn't. The programme is available free of charge from www.stammeringcentre.org.

The British Stammering Association (BSA)

Stammeringineducation.net is the British Stammering Association's online resource for teachers and school staff showing best practice for teachers and school staff when working with pupils who stammer, plus tips and techniques for English oral work. It includes video and audio clips of children who stammer, teachers and therapists, as well as classroom situations.

The Stuttering Foundation

The Stuttering Foundation provides free online resources, services and support to those who stutter, their families and professionals. Their website has information for teachers and they have produced a DVD and downloadable handbook, 'Stuttering: Straight Talk for Teachers'. There are information and resources for teachers at www.stutteringhelp.org.

Chapter 6

INFORMATION AND RESOURCES

There is help out there, but it's quite difficult to find. And it's difficult to find the right help.

Mother of 14-year-old boy

'Speech therapy is good. I feel a lot more open to speak because everyone there has got a stammer and they know what it's like and they understand what I'm going through and they try to help me as much as they can.'

Ndlovu, 9

Many children who stammer and their parents long for a 'cure'. When you type the word 'stammering' or 'stuttering' into a search engine, you will get a list of websites, some of which seem to offer a cure. You will also find the websites of self-help organisations and of speech and language therapists.

Speech and language therapists do not use the word 'cure'. Occasionally, a person who stammers finds a programme or a type of therapy that works for him, he sees it as a 'cure' and he may want to share his experience. However, it is important to remember that some of the 'therapies' that are offered are unregulated.

We would recommend that parents are cautious and gather information before signing up to these programmes. The websites of the British Stammering Association and the Stuttering Foundation (see Chapter 5) are a good source of information and advice.

HOW TO ACCESS THERAPY

'I think it would be useful to have some speech therapy coz it teaches you new techniques like how to cope with it and how to actually live with it and different ways of trying to control it.'

Waseem, 14

We know that the earlier a child receives help for stammering the more effective therapy can be, so try to refer your child to a speech and language therapist as soon as you can. This does not mean that older children and teenagers cannot be helped – they too should be referred, as therapy can be enormously helpful in giving them strategies to improve their fluency and in building their confidence.

There is a speech and language therapy service in most areas of the UK. Some areas have a 'direct access' policy, which means you can refer your child directly. You could call in at your local health centre for information about contacting the local speech and language therapist.

If there is no direct access policy, you can ask your family doctor or health visitor to refer you to your local speech and language therapy service. Some services hold drop-in clinics in health centres, and you don't need a referral for these. There are often waiting lists, so it is best to refer your child as soon as you have concerns. You can always let them know if he doesn't need to be seen when the appointment becomes available.

Once your child has been referred you may be offered a screening appointment quite quickly, when the speech and language therapist will decide what should happen next. You may be offered an assessment, which may or may not be followed by therapy, or you may be given advice and a review appointment in future. You may have to wait for these appointments.

Your child's school may be able to help too. Some have speech and language therapists who visit on a regular basis, or the head teacher may have a contact telephone number for someone in your area.

Sometimes parents are told that their child is too young to have speech and language therapy. If your child has a relative who stammers and your child's stammer is getting worse, we would advise against the 'wait and see' policy.

As stammering is a complex speech problem it is helpful to find a speech and language therapist who is experienced in the disorder. There is a specialist therapist in stammering in some areas and there are some specialist centres for the assessment and treatment of stammering.

Another option is to look for an independent speech and language therapist. To find one in your area, see the Association of Speech and Language Therapists in Independent Practice website www. helpwithtalking.com. Make sure you look for a therapist who specialises in 'stammering', 'stuttering' or 'dysfluency' in children.

The British Stammering Association has a helpline (0845 603 2001) or you can email info@stammering.org for information about finding your local speech and language therapist (in the UK).

The Stuttering Foundation has an international referral list of people who specialise in the treatment of stammering at www.stutteringhelp. org.

ASSESSMENT

'Therapy has been amazing. It's really helped me and because the speech therapists are used to people stammering, you don't feel you have to try to hide it and so when you do stammer they give you special techniques and stuff to help you.'

Billy, 11

A speech and language therapy assessment will differ depending on the age of the child.

In a preschool child we need to establish whether the dysfluency is a temporary phase, which the child is likely to grow out of naturally, or whether it is more likely to persist if left untreated. This assessment usually involves the parents giving information to the therapist to help determine what the most probable outcome is for their child. The therapist may not need to see the child. The questions that may be asked are listed below.

Questions that parents may be asked at a screening appointment for a young child who stammers

1. What does he do when he stammers?
   Does he repeat whole words, e.g. 'but but but'?
   Does he repeat parts of words, e.g. 'b-b-but'?
   Does he stretch out sounds, e.g. 'mmmmum'?
   Does he get stuck on a sound and nothing comes out?
   Does he do anything else with his face or body when he stammers?
   Does he give up on trying to say it?

2. Do you think he is aware of it? Do you think he is worried about it?

3. On a scale of 0 to 7, where 0 is 'normal' and 7 is 'very severe', how severe is the stammering?

4. When did he start stammering?

5. Has it changed since then? In what way?

6. When is it best and when is it worst?

7. On a scale of 0 to 7, where 0 is 'not at all worried' and 7 is 'extremely worried', where are you now?

8. If he is talking to you and he stammers, what do you do or say to try and help?

9. Has either parent ever stammered? Do they still?

10. Did any blood relative on either side of the family ever stammer? Do they still?

11. Does your child have any other speech or language difficulties now?

12. Has he had any other speech or language difficulties in the past?

13. Do you think his language skills are better than other children of his age?

14. Are there any other issues that we should be aware of?

In older children and teenagers the assessment typically involves a session with the child and a separate session with the parents. The aim of the assessment is to establish what the stammering is like, how frequent it is, how it affects the child and his family, and what factors may be contributing to it.

In the child assessment, the therapist evaluates the stammering – the type and frequency of the stammer, whether there are associated body movements, whether the child is aware of it and anything he does to manage it. A video recording may be made which the therapist can analyse.

The therapist will ask the child about his speech and discuss the impact of the stammer on his life. Questionnaires may be used that can be scored to give a measure of the severity of the stammer and its effect on the child and on his daily life.

We know that stammering can vary from day to day, and the child may hardly stammer when he comes for assessment. An experienced therapist will not send the family away on the strength of this. The parents and the child can describe what the stammer is like when it is more marked, and therapy decisions can be based on this information.

The assessment session with the parents involves taking a case history, which includes all the relevant background information. This can be more wide-ranging and detailed than typical case histories, as stammering is more complicated than other speech difficulties.

Some older teenagers choose not to have their parents involved in the assessment or therapy process.

Once the assessment has been completed, the findings are discussed with the parents and child (as appropriate). The therapist describes the options if therapy is recommended. There may be a waiting period, especially if intensive group therapy is involved, as groups are typically held during school holidays.

The therapist will write a report for the parents and family doctor and this will usually also be sent to the school and other people involved with the child, with the parents' consent.

WHAT TO EXPECT IN THERAPY

'After speech therapy it's fine. I put my hand up a lot more and I'm fine with speaking. It's a lot better and I feel that I've made a big improvement, I'm talking slower and not racing.'

Nazim, 10

Children under seven

There are two main therapy approaches for young children who stammer. Both have been researched to see how effective they are and, in general, four out of five children who receive early intervention will stop stammering.

PALIN PARENT–CHILD INTERACTION THERAPY

The therapy involves parents attending a weekly session with their child for six weeks.

Parents explore how they can help their child to be more fluent by talking and playing with the child and then watching video feedback. They practise this at home during five-minute 'special times'.

They also discuss how the whole family can help the child's speech, for instance when they are all together. After the six clinic sessions, the parents continue the therapy at home for another six weeks, followed by a review appointment in the clinic to discuss how the child is progressing.

Our research has shown that a child will usually begin to improve in the period following the six clinic sessions. If the child's speech has not improved by the review session, more therapy is offered, which involves working with the child to make small changes to his way of speaking which will help him be more fluent.

THE LIDCOMBE PROGRAM

Parents attend once-weekly sessions with their child.

The therapist shows the parent how to have structured talking times with the child when the parent will praise the child when he speaks fluently – for example, 'That was smooth talking.' Parents also give the child feedback when he stammers – for example, 'That was a bit bumpy,' although they are instructed to focus more on the fluent than the stammered speech.

This method has been shown to reduce stammering after an average of 11 therapy sessions.

School-age children

'In the second year of school, I kept on stammering and I couldn't get a word out and I went to speech therapy and they said, "Don't worry about a thing and don't let anything get in your way," and then I practised all the tools and it's coming together and I'm getting fluent.'

Adi, 10

Therapy with primary school-age children tends to combine helping parents and families make changes to support a child's fluency, together with individual work with the child.

The child and his parents may attend on their own or in a group. Many children who stammer tell us that they feel that they are 'the only person in the world who stammers', and groups can be really helpful if this is the case.

Groups are also the perfect setting for trying out new fluency and communication skills. Groups are held on a once-weekly basis or they may take place for a week or two weeks during term time or the school holidays.

Therapy has three strands: helping the child to control his stammering, working on his communication skills and building his confidence. These are described in some detail later in this chapter.

Teenagers

> 'I find speech therapy very helpful because at the moment I've got very bad speech but after some therapy I find it a lot easier coz all the things I've been taught on courses all come back to me and I get more fluent and it really does help me.'
>
> *Tom, 15*

It's after school you worry about, it's the future, it's job interviews. There could be half a dozen candidates but because of your speech you could be brushed aside, you could be at the bottom of the pile.

Father of 15-year-old boy

As a child reaches his teens there is less family involvement in the therapy. The components of therapy are described below and there may be additional activities to help students prepare for life beyond school.

For example, young people can practise interview skills for university or jobs. This involves more than just a focus on managing fluency – the student thinks about his communication skills as a whole, as well as what he is saying. Some students find that at the beginning of the interview it can be helpful to say something like, 'I may stammer today, but if you would just bear with me, I will get there in the end.'

Therapy may include working on telephone skills or any other situations that the student finds difficult because of his stammer.

Group therapy can be very helpful at this age but you may have to travel further afield to find it. The Michael Palin Centre runs groups for teenagers, and information about other group therapy programmes appears later in this section. Details of therapy available across the UK are updated on the British Stammering Association website.

COMPONENTS OF THERAPY

Speech control

> 'Everyone who stammers should come to speech therapy because it's really useful and I learned quite a lot of techniques and it just makes life easier for you.'
>
> Trisha, 9

The child may learn a speech technique, which usually involves speaking more slowly, with more pausing, flowing words together or softening some of the hard speech sounds.

At the Michael Palin Centre, we teach children how to do this using a video recording of a text being read aloud. It is read extremely slowly, with frequent pauses and with the words running into each other. This usually eliminates any stammering and the child practises at the extremely slow rate until he can do it easily. Then he gradually speeds up his speech to make it sound more natural. The children make video recordings of themselves to check their fluency and to listen to their speech.

Children can often do this quite easily, and they can use the technique in the clinic or when they are practising at home. It is much harder to keep using the technique for any length of time because it takes effort and concentration. Even when they are very skilled at it, and even though they might be very fluent, children tell us that it feels more natural when they go back to stammering.

Parents are often bewildered and frustrated by this – until we teach them the technique and ask them to use it in their daily lives. Once they discover how unfamiliar it feels and how much effort is involved in using the technique they understand why the child is not using it all the time.

We try to help the child use the technique outside the clinic environment by taking him out so that he can practise it in different situations. These may include buying things in shops or asking for directions under the supervision of the therapist.

We are often asked if we work on children's breathing, as stammering can interfere with natural breathing patterns. Children sometimes speak very quickly on one breath, often running out of air, for fear that if they stop to breathe they will get stuck. Or sometimes they speak on an in-breath, sounding rather strangulated. Sometimes, when they block on words, they sound as if they don't have enough air in their lungs.

We tend not to focus on breathing at the Michael Palin Centre. We find that if the child uses natural pauses and speaks more slowly, any breathing problems sort themselves out. Focusing on breathing can result in unnaturally deep breaths, which can have the undesired effect of building tension and sounding peculiar.

Communication skills

> Going on the course really made us look at things positively and we could see that if she used her techniques she could make a lot of progress. It really changed our lives for the better. Especially learning about praise, encouragement, taking turns. We used to give her too much time, we wrapped her up in cotton wool. 'No one speak while she is speaking!' It was terrible for the family.
>
> *Mother of 12-year-old girl*

In therapy we also focus on the child's social interaction skills, which can be affected by their stammer.

Children who opt out of talking in a group may need to work on taking turns in a conversation. Sometimes the opposite is the case – at home they may talk for too long as their parents were advised not to interrupt them.

Eye contact is very important because some children who stammer do not look at the person they are speaking to, maybe because they feel self-conscious.

Listening may have been affected by the stammering. The children learn how to show they are listening and how to focus on what is being said.

Body language may also be discussed – stammering can involve lots of tension resulting in body movements and fidgeting. Some children find that learning to sit comfortably and keep still may help their fluency.

An improvement in a child's general interaction skills can have a huge impact on his effectiveness as a communicator, even if he still stammers, so we believe it is essential to look at the child as a whole, rather than just focusing on the mouth.

Confidence building

'If someone said that I'm inferior to someone else because of my talking, then well obviously I disagree because at school I'd like to think I'm one of the bright ones, so if that's how they want to think, then fine by me.'

Joe, 15

Therapy will also include building the child's confidence, and we encourage the parents to praise the child more, and to help the child to view himself more positively.

We teach the child and his family problem-solving techniques to help them generate a range of solutions when they feel stuck. It is often a revelation for parents that their children can help them solve a problem by suggesting new ideas and ways to tackle it.

Parents learn that the child can cope with challenging situations and that he is capable of sorting things out for himself. We call this 'passing the ball back' and it can have an enormous effect on the child's confidence.

Therapy may also involve helping the child to 'mind less' about his stammer. Many children who stammer become very tuned into their speech and are acutely aware of every stumble and glitch. They are often very hard on themselves for stammering.

We try to help them feel a bit less sensitive about the times when they stammer. We can do this by letting them see themselves stammering in the mirror or on a video recording. Although this is difficult at first, they do get used to it and start to react less strongly. They also talk about their stammer, they stammer deliberately and teach others to stammer in the way that they do.

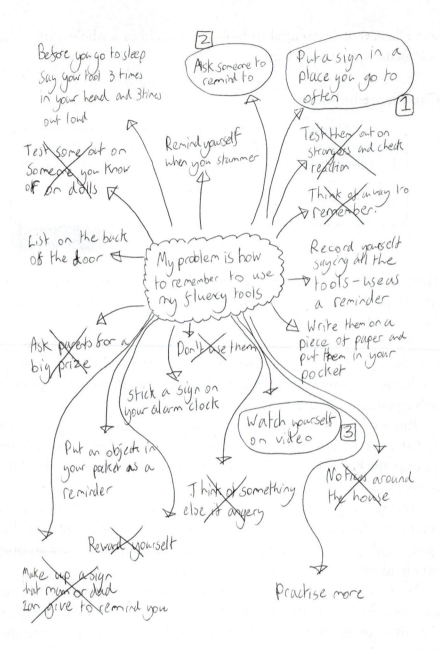

An example of problem solving in a children's group on 'How to remember to use my fluency tools'

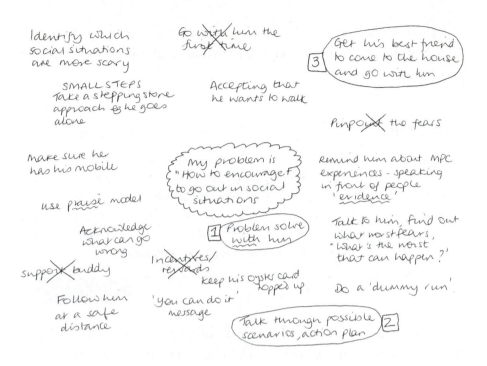

An example of problem solving in a parents' group on 'How to encourage a child to go out in social situations'

Children who stammer often think that everyone else is only noticing the stammer and they predict that people are making negative judgements about them. This mindset can affect their fluency. The way a child predicts reactions – 'They'll laugh at me' or 'I won't get picked for the team' – can increase his anxiety or embarrassment. This in turn can heighten physical tension, which can result in more stammering. Some children opt out of speaking altogether.

We help the child to observe other people's reactions when he does stammer, to see if his predictions always come true. This process gradually desensitises the child to his stammer, which makes him feel better and reduces the knock-on effects of the stammer.

We also want to foster a 'have a go' attitude, so that children are pleased with themselves for trying to do something, whatever the outcome. They learn to stretch their comfort zones, doing things that they might previously have avoided, like answering the phone or ordering their own meal in a restaurant. And if they stammer when they do it, they have still succeeded in the task. It's a win-win situation.

These confidence-building techniques may reduce the stammering, but they are also aimed at helping the child reach his potential in spite of his stammer.

RELAPSE

'Therapy is very important because without it I wouldn't have got where I am, coz before I came here I couldn't string together a sentence or two and now I can do it quite fluently. But when I go through a bad phase and I go to therapy it helps and I come out feeling more confident in myself and it shows.'

Jimmy, 16

With early intervention, many young children do very well in therapy and the stammer may disappear. In most cases, this fluency is life long and the stammer was a mere blip in the child's early development. However, in some cases the stammer emerges again at a later stage.

Similarly, older children may become much more fluent with therapy, to the extent that neither the child nor his parents are bothered about it any more and they agree with the therapist that they no longer need to attend. Some of these families get in touch with us later to say that the stammer is causing some concern and they would like more help.

So relapse seems to be a common phenomenon in stammering. Other speech problems tend not to relapse. A child who has unclear speech usually improves and his speech does not break down again. Similarly, a child whose language development is delayed tends to catch up with his peers and does not then regress.

At the Michael Palin Centre we have noticed over the years that there seem to be some critical times when a child is more likely to relapse. Starting at a new school or entering a new academic year with a new teacher can be a tricky time. Moving up to secondary school is especially challenging. It's a major transition from a small school with one class teacher to a much bigger building with many more pupils and different subject teachers in several classrooms. Teenagers can also find that their stammering increases when they start university or college or a new job.

It isn't hard to see why the stammering comes back or gets worse in these situations. We all wonder how we will cope and what others may think of us. Having a speech difficulty just adds a layer of anxiety to an already stressful situation.

Parents have also told us that less significant life events also trigger relapse. They say that fluency in young children can break down during major religious and public holidays. It may be that a change of environment and routine, different mealtimes and bedtimes, lack of sleep, being with different people and getting very excited all affect the child's fluency.

We have found that some therapy input at these times of relapse can help the child or teenager to get back on track. Very often they will just need to be reminded of the things that were beneficial before. Sometimes, additional techniques may be incorporated. It is certainly worthwhile to contact the therapist again to ask for advice or help.

OTHER TYPES OF THERAPY

'Some therapy was better than others. I think different things work for different people and you have to find what helps you and keep practising and then it gets better.'

Sarah, 16

Cognitive behaviour therapy (CBT)

Cognitive behaviour therapy is a form of psychological counselling, which is widely used in the treatment of anxiety and depression. There is lots of evidence that it is highly effective. Some speech and language therapists who specialise in stammering have also been trained in CBT, and therapy for stammering now has many components of CBT integrated into it.

CBT looks at the way our thoughts influence our feelings and our behaviour. If we think 'He thinks I'm stupid' this is likely to make us feel anxious or nervous which can affect us physically, making us go red or break out into a sweat. This then affects our behaviour, so we might stumble over words, stop talking or make a hasty exit. 'He thinks I'm stupid' is only what we imagine, it is not a fact, and if we walk away we may never find out whether it is true. This is called a 'vicious cycle'.

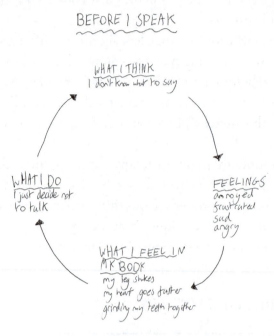

BEFORE I SPEAK

WHAT I THINK
I don't know what to say

WHAT I DO
I just decide not
to talk

FEELINGS
annoyed
frustrated
sad
angry

WHAT I FEEL IN
MY BODY
my leg shakes
my heart goes faster
grinding my teeth together

A vicious cycle

> 'If I think a teacher's going to ask me lots of questions I think I will stammer coz I get very nervous and then I stammer more and sometimes I grit my teeth and sometimes I go red.'
>
> Ahmed, 10

CBT is used in stammering therapy with children and teenagers to help them notice the kinds of thoughts they might be having and to look at how these thoughts affect them. Sometimes they are more aware of their emotions than their thoughts. They may be aware of feeling worried, but when we ask them 'And you feel worried that…?' they are able to identify what is going through their heads.

Here are some typical examples of thoughts they may have:

- I know I will stammer.

- I'm going to mess this up.

- They won't want to listen to me.

- They will laugh.

- He thinks I'm stupid.

These may be linked to some of the following emotions:

- anxiety

- nervousness

- embarrassment

- shame

- fear

- frustration.

These thoughts and feelings may then lead to various changes in the body, such as:

- fast heartbeat

- changes in breathing

- getting hot and sweaty

- shaking hands or knees.

This may then affect how they behave:

- speak faster

- stammer more

- stop talking

- walk away

- say, 'I don't know.'

CBT looks at the impact of this vicious cycle and helps the person to consider how different, more helpful thoughts might change what happens next. We look at the thoughts and explore how true they are by testing them out: 'Do people think I'm stupid? Maybe some people don't. I know I'm not stupid. I've got better grades than them anyway.'

Challenging their negative thoughts can help the young people when they next catch themselves thinking in that way.

We sometimes encourage them to conduct an experiment to test whether the thought they have is based on fact. For example, they may think, 'People will look away because I am stammering.' They can test this out by talking to lots of people and finding out how many look away and how many don't. They may be pleasantly surprised.

Solution-focused brief therapy

Solution-focused brief therapy is another form of counselling therapy that has influenced therapy for stammering. It involves identifying what a person is already doing to manage a problem and building on that strength.

Electronic devices

'I would say that it isn't a miracle cure and it doesn't work magic so people shouldn't get their hopes up too much. But it might help some people in some situations.'

Max, 20

For many years it has been known that interfering with the way in which a person who stammers hears his own voice can make his speech more fluent. There are commercially produced electronic devices that delay or distort the sound of the voice and play it back to the person through an earpiece. The delayed feedback sounds rather like a long-distance telephone conversation used to, with the voice sounding almost like an echo. The distorted feedback is also at a different pitch. Both of these modifications usually help the person who stammers to speak more slowly and more fluently.

The two devices most commonly used are the VoiceAmp, which is like an iPod with an earpiece (price in the region of £700–£1000), or the SpeechEasy, which is an in-ear device rather like a hearing aid (price in the region of £2500–£3000).

Some teenagers and adults who stammer have found these devices very useful in certain situations, for example if they have to make a speech or talk on the phone. The effect doesn't tend to last – once the device is removed the person usually stammers again.

Medication

Over the years a number of drug therapies have been trialled with adults who stammer. While some may improve fluency, there are typically other side effects. There is currently no medication that is recommended by professional bodies for use in stammering therapy.

Other therapies

We are often asked if we would recommend hypnotherapy, acupuncture or a range of other treatments. There is no current research into the effectiveness of these approaches for stammering. However, there can be no doubt that some individuals have found them very helpful, while others did not. We believe it is important to be cautious about anything labelled a 'cure' for stammering, but we would not want to discourage someone from trying out a therapy that may be helpful.

THERAPY CENTRES

City Lit (London)

This is an adult education centre, which offers group therapy sessions for students (over 18) and other adults who stammer. Courses include daytime intensive courses, evening courses and short workshops, and a well-developed follow-up programme to provide ongoing support. Details at www.citylit.ac.uk.

City University London

Four-day intensive courses are run during school holidays in April and July, with follow-up days at half-term. Up to 24 people are accepted on each course and are divided into two groups: one for 8 to 11-year-olds and the other for those aged 12 to 18 plus. The primary aim of the course is to reduce the anxiety and embarrassment associated with stammering and to increase confidence. They also try to improve communication skills and to reduce the severity of the stammer to a more comfortable level for both speaker and listener. The courses are free of charge. Details at www.city.ac.uk/health/public-clinics/compass-centre/stammering-clinic/instensive-courses-for-people-who-stammer.

The Fluency Trust (Swindon)

Five-day residential courses are based in an Outward Bound activity centre in Devon, with a one-day follow-up later in the year. 'Blockbusters' is the course for children aged 10 to 12 years, and 'Teens Challenge' is for 13- to 17-year-olds. Therapy aims to increase confidence in communication, help develop a positive attitude to speaking and decrease sensitivity to stammering. There is a charge, which may be paid by an NHS Trust. The Fluency Trust may also assist with funding. Details at www.thefluencytrust.org.uk.

The Michael Palin Centre for Stammering Children

Children are referred by speech and language therapists or by GPs from all over the UK. The centre is run by the Whittington Health National Health Service with the support of the charity Action for Stammering Children. There is a charitably funded consultation service, which offers free-of-charge specialist assessment, advice and treatment recommendations for each family. Your local speech and language therapist will attend the appointment too.

Most families will then have therapy near their home with a review appointment after approximately six months. However, if the agreed recommendations are not available locally – for example, an intensive group therapy course – other possibilities will be discussed, including therapy at the Michael Palin Centre. In this case, funding is sought from the child's local NHS provider or other sources, and a course of therapy is arranged. Details at www.stammeringcentre.org.

The Stammering Support Centre (Leeds)

The centre is provided by Leeds Community Healthcare NHS Trust Speech and Language Therapy service, supported by Yorkshire and Humber Primary Care Trusts, Action for Stammering Children, the British Stammering Association and the Department for Education. The Centre offers specialist speech and language therapy assessment and support for children, young people and adults who stammer. Referrals can be from any part of the UK.

There are a number of assessment and therapy packages, including parents' workshops for early stammering, and therapy groups that focus on developing self-esteem. Details at www.leedscommunityhealthcare. nhs.uk/stammeringsupportcentre.

OTHER USEFUL ORGANISATIONS
AND WEBSITES

UK

British Stammering Association

The British Stammering Association keeps a register of speech and language therapy services. It also has an advice line, leaflets, pamphlets, books and videos packed with information. Details at www.stammering. org.

Royal College of Speech and Language Therapists (RCSLT)

This is the professional body for speech and language therapists in the UK. It promotes research into the field of speech and language therapy, and better education and training of speech and language therapists. It also provides information for its members and the public about speech and language therapy. Details at www.rcslt.org

AUSTRALIA

Australian Speak Easy Association

Australian Speak Easy is a self-help organisation that provides support for people who stutter by holding weekly meetings in their respective metropolitan and rural locations. Groups meet regularly to work on fluency techniques, discuss individual stuttering problems and develop self-confidence through role-playing and public speaking. To assist with this, the Association works side by side with Speech Pathologists to help keep members up to date on the latest techniques and treatments including the technique of Smooth Speech. Details at www.speakeasy. org.au.

SOUTH AFRICA
Speak Easy South Africa

South African Speak Easy is a support group for people who stutter, their family members and friends. Meetings are used to discuss issues around stuttering, to share new ideas and experiences, discuss feelings and to practise one's speech techniques. Speak Easy was started by a group of people who stutter, their parents and speech therapists to address the issue of prevention and treatment of stuttering in South Africa through education, self-help groups and by enhancing the training and skills of Speech Therapists. Details at www.speakeasy.org.za.

USA
Friends: The National Association of Young People Who Stutter

Friends: The National Association of Young People who Stutter is the only national organisation dedicated solely to empowering young people who stutter and their families. Their mission is to provide support and education to children and teens who stutter, their families and clinicians. Friends is a non-profit, volunteer organisation whose members include the young people, their parents and siblings but also adults who stutter and Speech Language Pathologists that have a special interest in stuttering. Details at www.friendswhostutter.org.

National Stuttering Association

The National Stuttering Association is the largest self-help support organisation in the United States for people who stutter. Their mission is to bring hope and empowerment to children and adults who stutter, their families, and professionals through support, education, advocacy, and research. Details at www.nsastutter.org.

The Stuttering Foundation

The Stuttering Foundation provides free online resources, services and support to those who stutter and their families, as well as support for research into the causes of stuttering. They are the first and the largest non-profit charitable organisation in the world working toward the prevention and improved treatment of stuttering, reaching over a million people annually. They also offer extensive training programs on stuttering for professionals. Details at www.stutteringhelp.org.

The Stuttering Homepage

The Stuttering Homepage is dedicated to providing information about stuttering and other fluency disorders for both consumers and professionals who work with people who stutter. It includes information about research, therapy, support organisations, resources for professors who teach fluency disorders courses, materials for young people who stutter, and much more. Details at www.stutteringhomepage.com.

EUROPE

The European League of Stuttering Associations

European League of Stuttering Associations: ELSA is a trans-national, cross-cultural organisation. It extends the exchange-of-information network. It aims to lobby for people who stutter at a different level. Details at www.stuttering.ws.

INTERNATIONAL

International Stuttering Association

The International Stuttering Association's objective is to improve the conditions for children, adolescents and adults who stutter and parents of children who stutter in all countries, by sharing concepts and information about self-help and therapy methods, educating the general public, stimulating research, being an advocate, assisting in the founding of international working groups and by initiating public relations projects. Details at www.stutterisa.org.

CONCLUSION

The fact that you have bought and read this book demonstrates how much you want to help children and young people who stammer.

We hope that the information here, which we have gathered both from our own experience and from published research, will have helped you to understand what stammering is, what causes it and how it affects a child who stammers and his family.

In the book, children say how parents, families and teachers can help. They also say what they would rather we didn't do. While some of these suggestions can be easily put into practice, others present more of a challenge.

If you are the parent of a child who stammers, we hope to have dispelled any feelings of guilt you may have had that you may have done something to cause your child to stammer. You have not. The advice in this book is only intended to show how you may be able to help your child to overcome, to alleviate or to live more comfortably with his stammer. We hope that you will be able to select some ideas that fit for you and your child.

Above all, we hope that the many courageous children and young people who speak out in this book will be listened to, and that their words will create a greater understanding of stammering.

REFERENCES

Andrews, G., Hoddinott, S., Craig, A., Howie, P., Feyer, A.M. and Neilson, M. (1983) 'Stuttering: A review of research findings and theories circa 1982.' *Journal of Speech and Hearing Disorders 48*, 226–246.

Beal, D.S. (2011) 'The advancement of neuroimaging research investigating developmental stuttering.' *Perspectives on Fluency and Fluency Disorders 21*, 3, 88–95.

Bernstein Ratner, N. (2010) 'Translating recent research into meaningful clinical practice.' *Seminars in Speech and Language 31*, 4, 236–249.

Bloodstein, O. and Ratner, N. (2008) *A Handbook on Stuttering*. Clifton Park, NY: Thomson/Delmar Learning.

Compton, D. (1993) *Stammering: Its Nature, History, Causes and Cures*. London: Hodder and Stroughton.

Coulter, C., Anderson, J. and Conture, E. (2009) 'Childhood stuttering and dissociations across linguistic domains: a replication and extension. *Journal of Fluency Disorders 34*, 4, 257–278.

Kang, C., Riazuddin, S. and Mundorff, J. (2010) 'Mutations in the lysosomal enzyme-targeting pathway and persistent stuttering.' *New England Journal of Medicine 362*, 8, 677–685.

Yairi, E. and Ambrose, N. (2005) *Early Childhood Stuttering: For Clinicians, by Clinicians*. Austin, TX: Pro-Ed.

INDEX